AF710408

Contraction and Relaxation in the Myocardium

Contraction and Relaxation in the Myocardium

Edited by

Winifred G. Nayler

Cardiothoracic Institute, London University, U.K.

ACADEMIC PRESS

London New York San Francisco

A Subsidiary of Harcourt Brace Jovanovich, Publishers

QP
113.2
.C66

ACADEMIC PRESS INC. (LONDON) LTD.
24/28 Oval Road,
London NW1

United States Edition published by
ACADEMIC PRESS INC.
111 Fifth Avenue
New York, New York 10003

Copyright © 1975 by
ACADEMIC PRESS INC. (LONDON) LTD.

All Rights Reserved
No part of this book may be reproduced in any form by photostat, microfilm, or any other means, without written permission from the publishers

Library of Congress Catalog Card Number 75-21612
ISBN: 0-12-514650-7

Printed in Great Britain by
Whitstable Litho Ltd., Whitstable, Kent.

Contributors

Barrett, Professor A.M., B.Pharm., Ph.D. Professor of Pharmacology, Department of Pharmacology, University of Leeds, Leeds, U.K.

Linden, Professor R.J., M.B., C.H.B., F.R.C.P., Ph.D., D.Sc. Professor of Cardiovascular Studies, Cardiovascular Unit, University of Leeds, Leeds, U.K.

Nayler, Winifred G., D.Sc. Cardiothoracic Institute, London University, U.K.

Noble, D., B.Sc., D.Phil. University Department of Physiology, Oxford, U.K.

Noble, M.I.M., M.D., M.B.BS., M.R.C.P. Midhurst Medical Research Institute, Midhurst, Sussex, U.K.

Perry, Professor S.V., B.Sc., Ph.D., Sc.D (Cantab.). Department of Biochemistry, University of Birmingham, Birmingham, U.K.

Pollack, G.H. Midhurst Medical Research Institute, Midhurst, Sussex, U.K. and Departments of Anesthesia and Bioengineering, University of Washington, Seattle, Washington, U.S.A.

Vaughan Williams, E.M., D.M., D.Sc., M.A. Department of Pharmacology, Oxford University, Oxford, U.K.

Wollenberger, Professor A., Ph.D., D.Sc., Bereichsdirektor am Zentralinstitut für Herz- und Kreislauf Regulationsforschung der Akademie der Wissenschaften der DDR Berlin-Buch, D.D.R.

Preface

Whether we be biochemists, physiologists, pharmacologists or cardiologists we all share one thing in common - namely, the continual exposition of new findings and data relating to our own particular field of study. Beleiving that it is the comprehension of such newly acquired data which provides the stimulus not only for further research but also for the re-consideration and re-evaluation of our currently accepted theories and hypotheses, a short intensive course entitled "The Scientific Basis of Cardiology" was organised by the Institute of Cardiology in London. This course was held during 1974, and two days of it was devoted to discussions relating to the events which regulate the cyclic sequence of contraction and relaxation in heart muscle. The formal papers presented during these discussions form the bases of this book. In compiling these papers the authors, all of whom are recognized authorities in their own particular fields of study, were asked to prepare authoritive reviews of their subjects and to present them in such a way as to provide not only interesting and easily read chapters, but also a valuable source of reference. I am sure that the individual authors have achieved this objective, and that many of the findings which are documented here will provoke further discussion, interest and research.

PREFACE

We are all deeply indebted to Merck Sharp & Dohme Ltd. (Great Britain) who so generously financed and supported this meeting.

My own sincere thanks are due not only to the contributors to this volume but also to Miss Martin and Judy Stephenson who have helped with the preparation of the final manuscripts.

WINIFRED G. NAYLER

Contents

The Cardiac Cell

WINIFRED G. NAYLER

Cardiothoracic Institute, London University, U.K.

Although there is now substantial support for the view that the transition from the resting to the active state in heart muscle cells is regulated by phasic changes in the intracellular availability of ionized calcium (Katz, 1971) and despite our increased understanding of the way in which these ions interact with the contractile elements (Perry, 1975), the biochemical basis of the link between excitation and the mechanical response remains obscure. Whilst it is known that depolarization of the cell membrane beyond a critical level is accompanied by an inwards displacement of calcium from the extra- to the intracellular phase (Reuter and Beeler, 1969; Wood, Heppner and Weidmann, 1969) and that the activation of the mechanical response is strongly dependent upon this influx (Nayler and Merrillees, 1971), controversy does exist, as to whether sufficient Ca^{2+} is displaced inwards across the depolarization membrane to directly activate (Langer, Frank and Tellisch, 1974) the mechanical response. Alternatively, and as is shown schematically in Figure 1, those calcium ions which are displaced inwards across the depolarized cell membrane may trigger a release of additional calcium

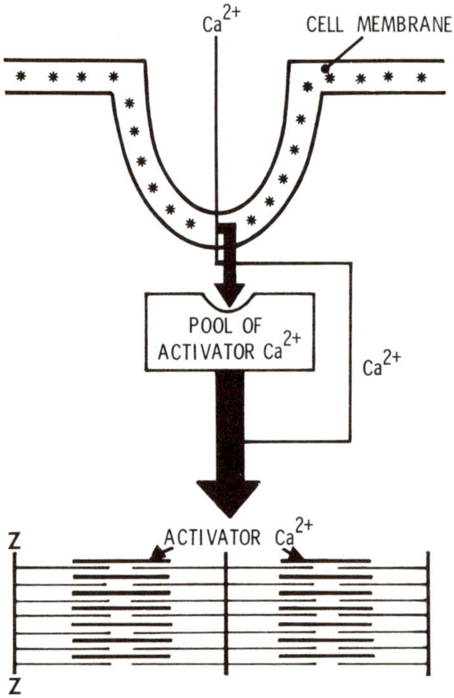

FIG. 1 Schematic representation of the inwards displacement of Ca^{2+} across a cardiac cell membrane and its possible role as a "trigger" to release additional Ca^{2+} from intracellular storage sites.

from intracellular storage sites (Nayler, 1966; Reuter and Beeler, 1969; Wood, Heppner and Weidmann, 1969; Nayler and Merrillees, 1971; Nayler and Dunnett, 1974; Bailey and Ong, 1974), and it may be these ions that activate the mechanical response.

Just as the activation of contraction depends upon the concentration of ionized calcium in the immediate vicinity of the myofibrils (Figure 2) exceeding a critical level (Weber, Herz and Reiss, 1964) so the transition from the active to the resting state depends upon a sudden reduction in

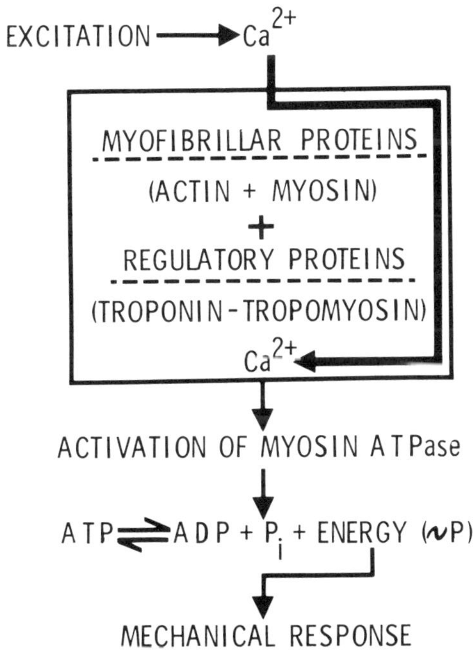

FIG. 2 Schematic representation of the events associated with excitation-contraction coupling in cardiac muscle.

their intracellular availability (Hasselbach and Makinose, 1961; Katz, 1971; Schwartz, 1971). This reduction in the intracellular availability of ionized calcium is almost certainly achieved via the intracellular sequestration of these ions (Hasselbach and Makinose, 1963), followed by the return of some of them to the extracellular phase. This retrieval of calcium from the immediate vicinity of the myofilaments, its possible storage for release in response to the arrival of another packet of "trigger-Ca^{2+}", and the return of some of it to the extracellular phase demands the presence not only of energy (as adenosine triphosphate) but also of appropriately located morphological structures which are capable of accumulating and exchanging calcium. An understanding of the way in which working heart muscle cells function at a subcellular level to facilitate either contraction or relaxation depends therefore, in part at least, upon an appreciation of the fine morphology of those cells. The various organelles which occur in a heart muscle cell have, for convenience, been listed in Table 1.

Because the first two components of this table – i.e. the contractile (actin and myosin) and regulatory (troponin 1, 11 + 11, and tropomyosin) proteins are discussed in detail in the second chapter of this book there is no need for us to refer to them in detail here. Instead it is sufficient to note that in cardiac as in skeletal muscle cells the fundamental unit of contraction is the sarcomere, the sarcomere being defined as the distance between two adjacent Z bands (Figure 1). Within each sarcomere the contractile

Table 1. Structure - function relationship of intracellular organelles in heart muscle.

SUBCELLULAR STRUCTURE	FUNCTION
CONTRACTILE PROTEINS (ACTIN AND MYOSIN)	CONTRACTION - RELAXATION
REGULATORY PROTEINS (TROPONIN AND TROPOMYOSIN)	Ca^{2+} SENSITIVITY
PLASMA MEMBRANE AND T - SYSTEM	DISTRIBUTION OF DEPOLARIZING CURRENT ? SUPPLY OF ACTIVATOR
SARCOPLASMIC RETICULUM	? SUPPLY OF ACTIVATOR Ca^{2+} SEQUESTRATION OF Ca^{2+} -> RELAXATION
MITOCHONDRIA	SUPPLY OF ~ ENERGY (ATP)
NUCLEUS, RIBOSOMES, LYSOSOMES etc.	CELL MAINTENANCE AND REGENERATION

proteins – actin and myosin – are arranged in an orderly but interdigitating array. Contraction involves a regulated displacement of the actin relative to the myosin filaments, a displacement which probably involves the formation of cross-bridges or linkages, between adjacent actin and myosin filaments. The energy required for the activation of these cross-bridges is derived from the hydrolysis of ATP (Mommaerts, 1974) and the relevant ATPase enzyme is associated with the myosin filament. In the resting state – i.e. when the myoplasmic concentration of Ca^{2+} is less than 10^{-7} M (Hasselbach and Makinose, 1961; Weber, 1966) the activity of this ATPase enzyme is inhibited by virtue of its interaction with the troponin complex (Hartshorne and Mueller, 1968, and Chapter 2). An increase in the intracellular availability of Ca^{2+} is associated with an increased binding of Ca^{2+} to the high affinity binding sites on a subunit of the troponin complex (Ebashi, Endo and Ohtsuki, 1969). The resultant conformational change results in the suppression of an inhibitory influence which the Ca^{2+}-depleted troponin complex exerts on the myosin ATPase enzyme (Ebashi and Endo, 1968). Now, if contraction within each cell is to be uniform and regular not only must the concentration of Ca^{2+} within that cell exceed the critical level of 10^{-7}M, but the distribution of that Ca^{2+} throughout the myoplasm must be fairly uniform with respect to the myofilaments. To understand how this uniformity might be achieved we must consider the morphology and distribution of the cell wall, because it is across this structure that calcium ions are displaced (Figure 3) inwards in response to the arrival of an excitatory stimulus.

THE CELL WALL

Cardiac muscle cells have a complex cell wall made up of

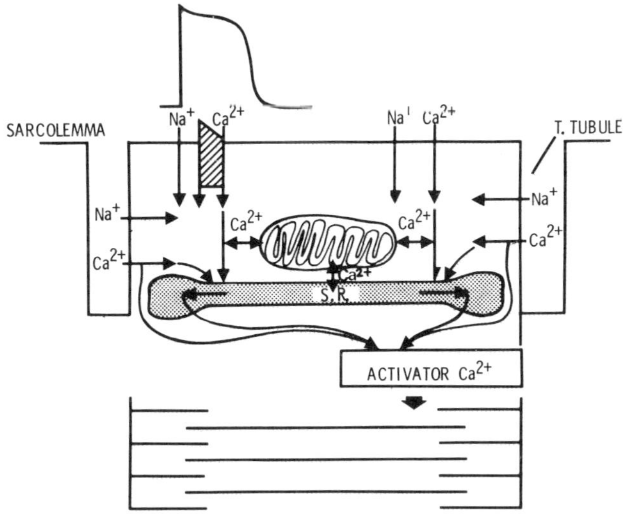

FIG. 3 Schematic representation of the relationship between the plasma membrane at the level of the sarcolemma and the sarcoplasmic reticulum as a source of "activator Ca^{2+}" for involvement in the sequence of events shown schematically in Figure 2.

(a) a plasma membrane, which is contiguous with the cytoplasm (Figures 4 and 5) and which often (Figure 5) exhibits marked pinocytotic activity,

(b) an extracellular protein-polysaccharide coating – the basement coat (Figures 4 and 5) and

(c) on the outermost surface, a diffuse reticulum of collagen fibrils.

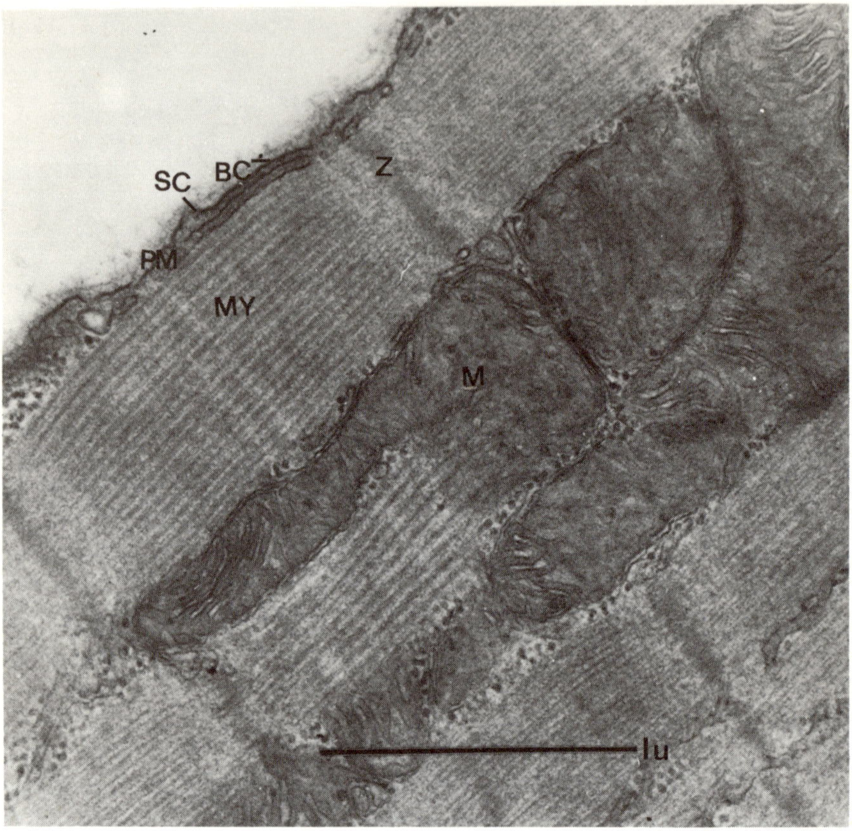

FIG. 4 Longitudinal section of guinea-pig papillary muscle (perfusion-fixed). Note presence of basement coat (B.C.), plasma membrane (P.M.), subsarcolemmal cisternae (S.C.) - forming part of the sarcoplasmic reticulum. My, myofilaments; M, mitochondria; Z, Z band.

The Plasma Membrane and the Basement Coat

The plasma membrane is between 8-9 nm thick. It is enzymatically

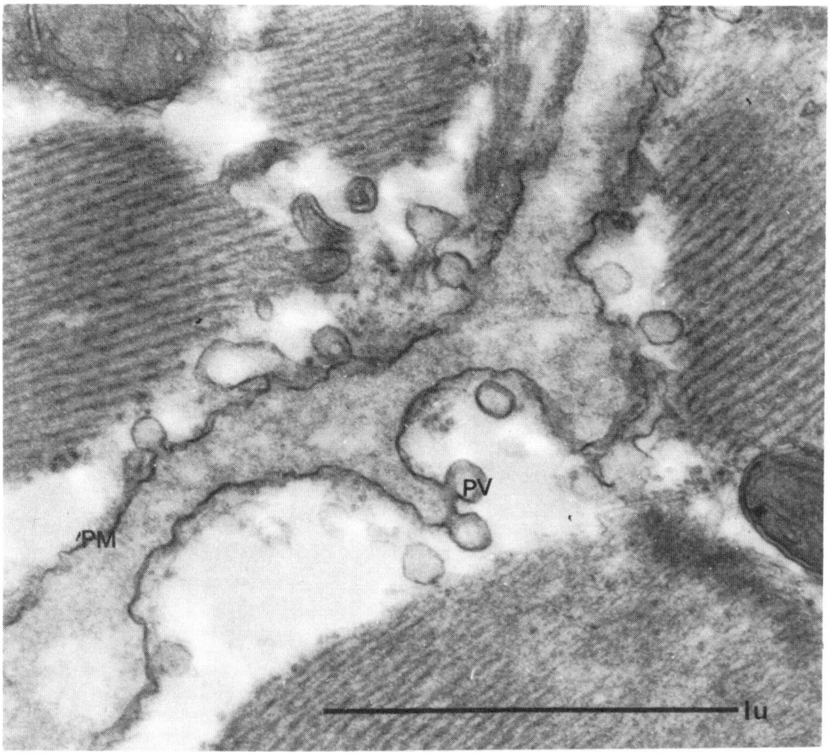

FIG. 5 Longitudinal section of perfusion-fixed frog ventricular muscle, showing marked pinocytotic activity of the plasma membrane (P.M.).

active, containing both $Na^{+}K^{+}$-activated (Schwartz, Lindenmayer and Allen, 1972) and Ca^{2+}-activated ATPase enzymes (Dietze and Hepp, 1971). Except where two cells abut end to end (Figure 6) the plasma membrane is covered by a layer of electron-dense, polysaccharide-like material which forms the basement coat. Until relatively recently the possible significance

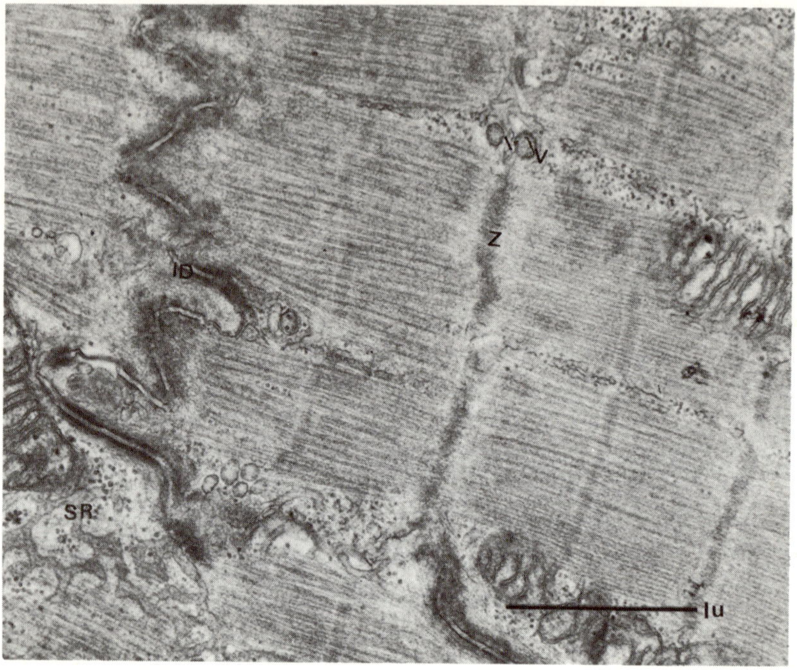

FIG. 6 Longitudinal section of perfusion-fixed guinea-pig heart muscle, showing specialized junction (the intercalated disc) between two adjacent cells.

of this basement coat layer as a reservoir or "trap" for Ca^{2+} (Figure 1) was overlooked. However, by using lanthanium (La^{3+}) to displace Ca^{2+} from this basement coat layer Langer and his colleagues (Langer and Frank, 1972) and others (Nayler and Merrillees, 1971; Nayler, 1973) have shown that this basement coat layer probably contains "an important fraction of the Ca^{2}" which is involved in excitation-contraction coupling in heart muscle cells".

The amount of calcium which is located within the basement coat layer will depend upon the number of fixed negatively charged sites which are available within the structure. According to Langer and his colleagues the Ca^{2+}-accumulating activity of these sites may be specifically attributable to their sialic acid content.

Whereas the plasma membrane is only 8-9 nm thick, the basement coat is much thicker. In cat ventricular muscle cells, for example, it is approximately 500 Å thick (Fawcett and McNutt, 1969) and can be further subdivided into a 200 Å thick inner and a 300 Å thick outer zone. Often the outer zone is more osmophillic than the inner layer (Fawcett and Selby, 1959).

Whilst the distribution of the basement coat layer is restricted to that of the plasma membrane, the distribution of the plasma membrane is not restricted to the periphery of the cell because tubular invaginations (Figures 7 and 8) of the plasma membrane extend into the cytoplasm, forming the transverse-tubular system. Experiments with electron-dense markers, e.g. colloidal lanthanum, horseradish peroxidase, and ferritin (Huxley, 1965; Forssmann and Girardier, 1970; Nayler and Merrillees, 1971) have shown unequivocally that the lumen of these tubules is continuous with that of the extracellular space, and that these tubules branch and ramify in all directions (Nayler and Merrillees, 1971). Usually these tubular invaginations occur at the level of the Z band.

The plasma membrane which lines these tubules is continuous with that of the periphery of the cell, and their lumen is filled with electron-dense basement coat material indistinguishable from that found at the periphery of the cell. Hence these tubular invaginations provide a mechanism for increasing the ratio between the surface area and the volume of the cell relative to that which would exist if the surface of the cell did not invaginate. Accordingly these tubules probably facilitate the rapid distribution of the excitatory stimulus throughout the cell, as well as providing a relatively large area for the exchange of metabolic substrates and of ions. However, whilst the existence of such tubular ramifications of the cell wall may facilitate the inwards distribution of the excitatory stimulus (Bastian and Nakajima, 1974) their existence cannot be essential to the functioning of heart muscle because some cardiac muscle cells are devoid of them. For example toad ventricular (Nayler and Merrillees, 1964), turtle atrium (Fawcett and Selby, 1958), chicken and humming bird (Sommer et al., 1972) and some atrial cells in the cat (Fawcett and McNutt, 1969) are without a T-system. Some authors have suggested that the absence of T-tubules might be correlated with the size of the cells, relatively small cells being devoid of such tubules. A careful examination of the relevant literature indicates, however, that the presence or absence of T-tubules does not correlate perfectly with cell size (Nayler, 1975). Because of their extensive branching and ramification it is difficult to assign a meaningful value to the diameter of T-tubules. If, however, the diameter of the tubule at the periphery of the cell us used as a guide, then (Table 2) we find that the diameter of T-tubules in heart muscle cells greatly exceeds that found in skeletal muscle. The T-tubules often approach close to mitochondria and although this relationship could provide an obvious advantage when considered in terms of the distance metabolic substrates must diffuse before reaching a mitochondrion a morphological structure linking the lining wall of the T-tubule and that of the mitochondria has not yet been established.

Table 2. Diameter of T - tubule opening in skeletal and cardiac muscle.

SPECIES	MUSCLE	DIAMETER
Skeletal Muscle		Å
RANA PIPIENS	SARTORIUS	260
" "	"	210-240
RANA TEMPORARIA	TWITCH	300
" "	SLOW	300
TOAD FISH	SWIM BLADDER	300
EPTESICUS FUSCUS) MYOTIS LUCIFUGUS)	CRICOTHYROID	300-400
CARDIAC MUSCLE		
FERRET	VENTRICULAR	500-800
HUMAN	PAPILLARY	1500
CAT	PAPILLARY	2500
RAT	PAPILLARY	2000-2500

Although the plasma membrane which defines the free surface of the cell displays intense pinocytotic activity, irrespective of species, such activity is not commonly found at the boundaries of two abutting cells, where the plasma membrane assumes the specialized configuration of the intercalated disc (Figure 6). Even when the plasma membrane invaginates into the cell to form a T-tubule (Figures 7 and 8) pinocytotic activity is evident in the plasma membrane lining that tubule (Figure 7). Obviously the increase in total area of the plasma membrane which occurs because of the formation of these pinocytotic vesicles makes the calculation of surface area to cell volume ratios a particularly difficult and perhaps hazardous procedure. In addition to the amphora-like vesicles which bud off from the plasma membrane, probably as the result of its pinocytotic activity, a second type of vesicle is found in association with the cell membrane (Simpson, Rayns and Ledingham, 1974). These are the "bristle-coated vesicles" (McNutt and Fawcett, 1969) which are sometimes seen budding off from the plasma membrane (Figure 7). The function of these bristle-coated vesicles has not as yet been clearly established, although they may be concerned with the metabolism and uptake of protein (Simpson et al., 1974).

THE SARCOPLASMIC RETICULUM

The sarcoplasmic reticulum (Franzini-Armstrong and Porter, 1964; Peachey, 1965; Martonosi, 1972) consists of an intricate, three dimensional lace-like network of branching and anastomosing tubules (Figure 9) which approach close to the plasma membrane (Figure 4), extend from one sarcomere to the next, and envelop the myofibrils. When isolated as a microsomal fraction fragments of this reticulum are able to accumulate Ca^{2+} against a concentration gradient (Martonosi, 1972) the rate of Ca^{2+}- accumulation being dependent in part at least, upon the rate of hydrolysis of ATP (Makinose and Hasselbach, 1965).

In marked contrast to the direct continuity which exists between the lumen of the T-tubule and that of the extracellular space, the lumen of the sarcoplasmic reticulum lacks this continuity with the extracellular phase – i.e. it is an intracellular organelle (Nayler and Merrillees, 1971; Forssmann and Girardier, 1970). Within this subcellular organelle, however, there is abundant evidence of specialization, so much so that the reticulum must be regarded as a heterogeneous structure.

Whenever the network of branching and anastomosing tubules encircles the myofilaments (Figure 9) it presents the appearance of a relatively thin, single-walled tubule. When, however, the reticulum approaches the plasma membrane, irrespective of whether this occurs at the periphery of the cell (Figure 4) or along the profiles of a T-tubule (Figures 7, 8 and 11) specialized "junctional areas" are found. These junctional areas include

(a) the facing membranes of the sarcoplasmic reticulum and the plasma membrane;

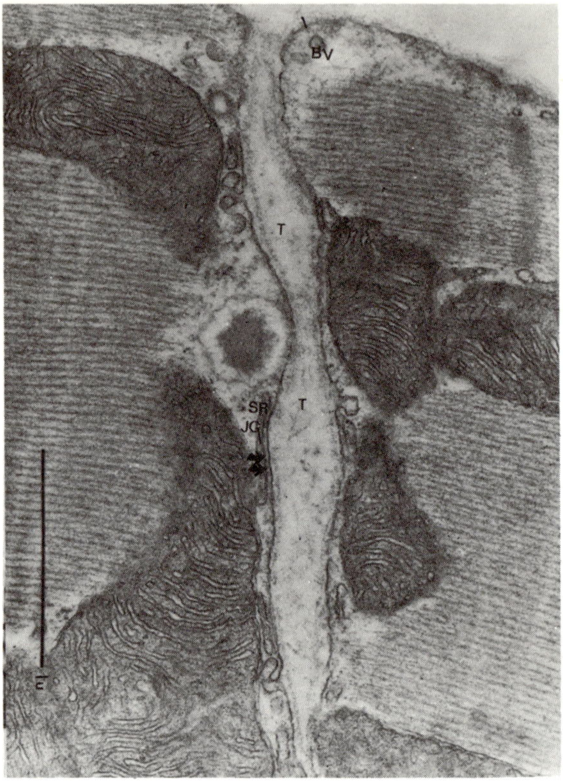

FIG. 7 Longitudinal section of perfusion-fixed rabbit papillary muscle, showing T-tubule invaginating from the cell membrane. Note that basement coat material fills the T-tubule. The walls of the tubule exhibit pinocytotic activity. B.V.: bristle coated vesicle. S.R.: part of the plasma membrane lying alongside the T-tubule. Note the electron-dense feet (arrows) protruding from the wall of the S.R. into the junctional gap (see text) whic

(b) an intervening gap, which is approximately 200 Å wide;

(c) regularly arranged electron-dense feet which project from the facing membranes of the sarcoplasmic reticulum (Figures 8, 10 and 11). These electron-dense feet are approximately 150 Å long. They are arranged in rows and although the presently available electron micrographs have failed to provide evidence of a direct continuity across the junctional gap, it is possible that the missing 50 Å is occupied by a structure which is not electron-dense. Electron-dense feet are spaced at regular intervals, protruding from the wall of the sarcoplasmic reticulum and extending into the junctional gap. These structures have been described in detail elsewhere (Nayler, 1975; Franzini-Armstrong, 1973), and despite their identification their possible function remains a mystery. Because similar electron-dense feet are found at the peripheral couplings (Figures 4 and 10) it is tempting to suggest that they may facilitate the direct transfer of information from the plasma membrane to the sarcoplasmic reticulum or vice versa. Could these structures facilitate the transfer of the electrical signal from the plasma membrane to the sarcoplasmic reticulum, or do they facilitate the exchange of ions, including Ca^{2+}? Such an exchange of

---

separates the lining membrane of the S.R. from that of the T-tubule. Junctional granules are located within this part of the S.R.

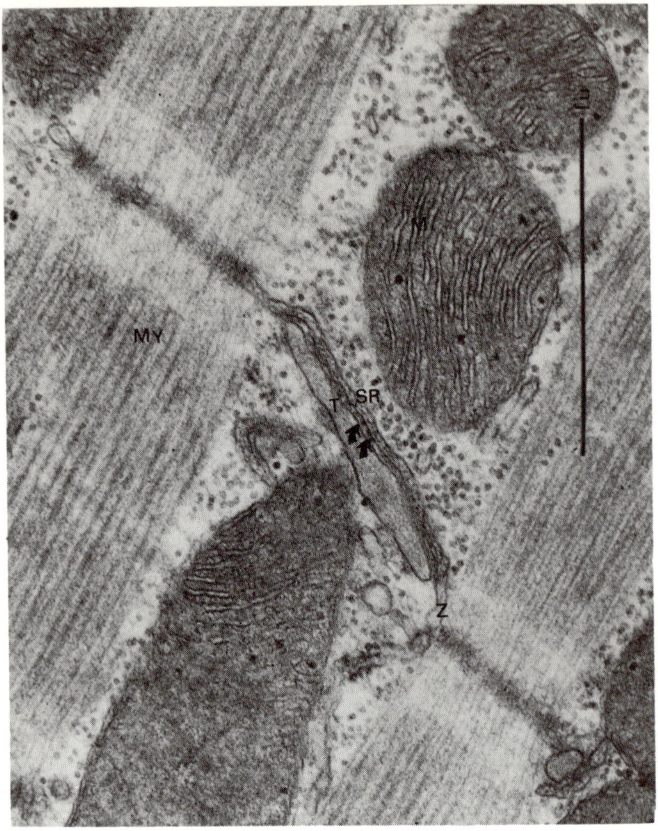

FIG. 8 Longitudinal section of perfusion-fixed guinea-pig papillary muscle showing specialized relationship between the T-tubule (T) and junctional sarcoplasmic reticulum. Note presence of granules in the lumen of the S.R., and electron-dense feet in the junctional gap which separates the lining wall of the T-tubule from that of the S.R. Z, Z-tubule, located at the level of the Z band.

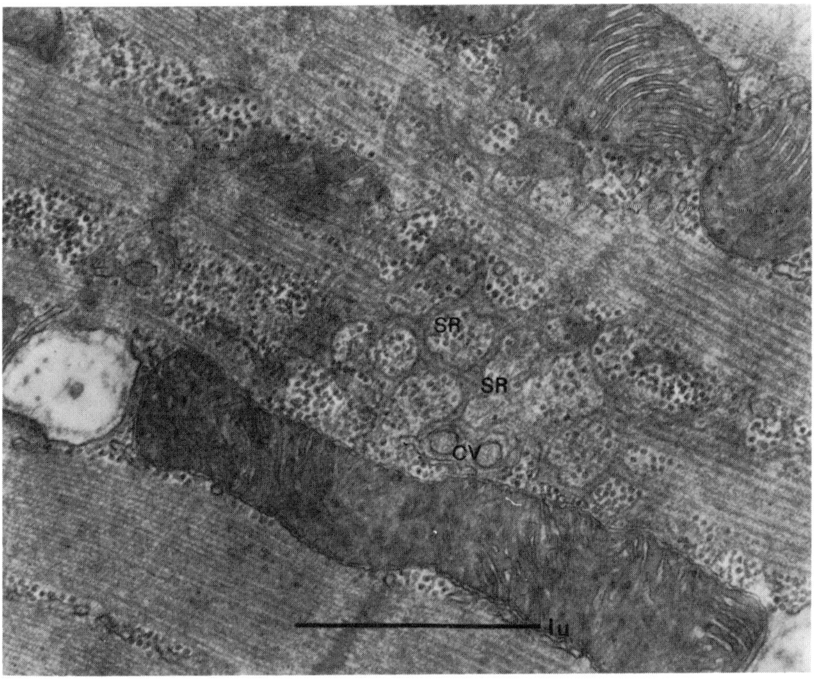

FIG. 9 Longitudinal section of perfusion-fixed guinea-pig papillary muscle showing lace-like distribution of the sarcoplasmic reticulum wrapping around the myofibrils, and the specialization of the reticulum (S.R.) alongside the T-tubule (T). Note presence of coated vesicles (C.V.).

ions could be bidirectional facilitating the bidirectional exchange of ions needed to account for the influx of Ca^{2+} during excitation, and the return of that Ca^{2+} to the extracellular phase during relaxation. Can it be that the specialization which exists within the sarcoplasmic reticulum is

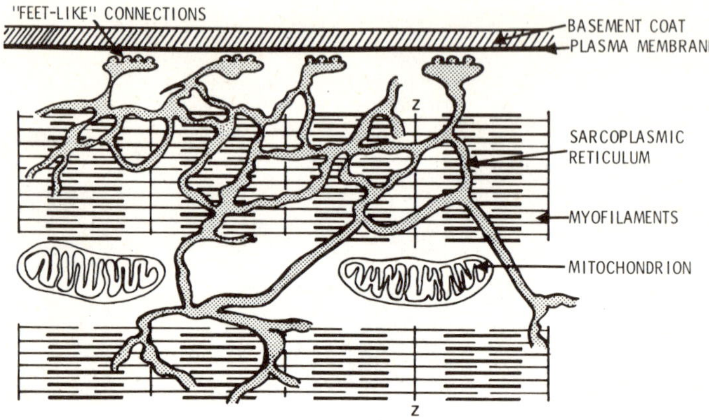

FIG. 10 Schematic representation of the special relationship between the S.R. and the cell wall, with "feet-like" structures protruding from the S.R. and pointing towards the plasma membrane (compare with electron micrograph in Figure 4).

accountable for in terms of a part of the reticulum which has developed to handle the trigger Ca^{2+}, and another part, closely associated with the myofilaments, and which has developed to supply and then sequester Ca^{2+} from the myofilaments? Clearly, although the techniques which have been developed to study the manner in which the reticulum accumulates and releases Ca^{2+} have provided us with valuable data concerning the biochemistry of this system they have, by destroying the delicate specialization which exists in the in vivo state, confused our understanding of the way in which this system regulates the intracellular availability of Ca^{2+},

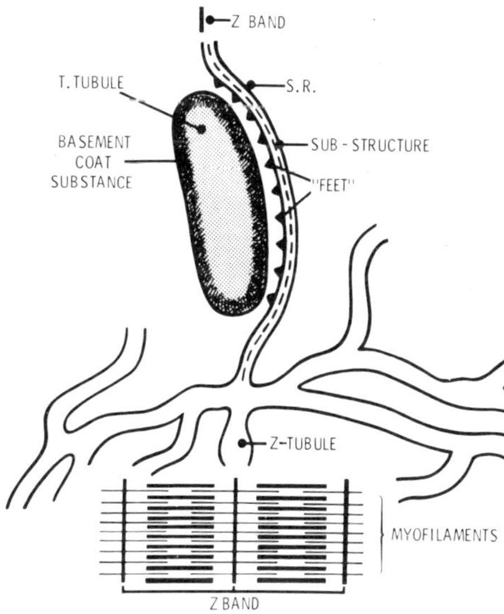

FIG. 11 Schematic representation of the relationship between the S.R. and T-tubule, showing specialized section of S.R., with attached electron-dense feet and intraluminal granules. These specialized parts of the reticulum apparently communicate with a Z-tubular portion of the reticulum.

to facilitate contraction and relaxation. It is not only the fine morphology of these functional couplings which are destroyed as the result of the currently used techniques of homogenization and differential centrifugation. Other specialized structures – e.g. the dense-coated vesicles (Figures 6 and 9) which are found in association with that part of the reticulum which envelops the myofilaments are lost from the system.

(d) the fourth component of this specialized function is found within the lumen of the reticulum, because here we find electron-dense granules. These electron-dense "junctional granules" are found only within that part of the sarcoplasmic reticulum which approaches close to the plasma membrane, irrespective of whether this involves the plasma membrane at the periphery of the cell – i.e. a "peripheral coupling" (Sommer and Johnson, 1969) or along a T-tubule. An example of such a coupling at the level of a Z band is shown in Figures 7 and 8. Here we can see that the sarcoplasmic reticulum which runs parallel to the plasma membrane contains an intraluminal structure, consisting of an array of granules. Once again we must ask ourselves what does this specialization which occurs with the sarcoplasmic reticulum mean, and is the specialization related to the close proximity of the plasma membrane?

Acknowledgement: This work was supported by the British Heart Foundation and the Medical Research Council of Great Britain.

REFERENCES

Bailey, L.E. and Ong, S.D. (1974). Calcium pools in excitation-contraction coupling in the cat heart: in ed. N. S. Dhalla and G. Rona. Myocardial Biology, 4, 255. University Park Press, London.

Bastian, J. and Nakajima, S. (1974). Action potential in the transverse tubules and its role in the activation of skeletal muscle. J. Gen. Physiol., 63, 257.

Dietze, G. and Hepp, K.D. (1971). Calcium-stimulated ATP-ase of cardiac sarcolemma. Biochem. Biophys. Res. Comm., 44, 1041.

Ebashi, S. and Endo, M. (1968). Calcium ion and muscle contraction. Progr. Biophys. Molec. Biol., 18, 123.

Ebashi, S., Endo, M. and Ohtsuki, I. (1969). Control of muscle contraction. Quart. Rev. Biophys., 2, 351.

Fawcett, D.W. and McNutt, N.S. (1969). The ultrastructure of the cat myocardium. Ventricular papillary muscle. J. Cell. Biol., 42, 1.

Fawcett, D.W. and Selby, C. (1958). Observations on the fine structure of the turtle atrium. J. Biophys. Biochem., 4, 63.

Forssmann, W.G. and Girardier, L. (1970. A study of the T systems in rat heart. J. Cell. Biol., 44, 1.

Franzini-Armstrong, C. (1973). Studies of the triads. Structure of the junction in frog slow fibers. J. Cell. Biol., 56, 120.

Franzini-Armstrong, C. and Porter, K.R. (1964). Sarcolemmal invaginations constituting the T system in fish muscle fibers. J. Cell. Biol., 22, 657.

Hartshorne, D.J. and Mueller, H. (1963). Fractionation of troponin into two distinct proteins. Biochem. Biophys. Res. Comm., 31, 647.

Hasselbach, W. and Makinose, M. (1961). Die Calciumpumpe der "Erschlaffungsgrana" des Muskels und ihre AbhaengigKeit von der ATP-Spaltung. Biochem., 2, 333, 159.

Hasselbach, W. and Makinose, M. (1963). Über den Mechanismus des Calcium transportes durch die Membranen des sarcoplasmatischen Retikulum. Biochem., 2, 345, 159.

Huxley, H.E. (1965). Structural evidence concerning the mechanism of contraction in striated muscle. In "Muscle" eds. Paul, Daniel, Kay and Monckton, p.3. Pergamon Press, London.

Katz, A.M. (1971). Calcium and the cardiac contractile proteins. In "Calcium and the Heart" p.124. Eds. Harris and Opie. Academic Press, London.

Langer, G.A. and Frank, J.S. (1972). Lanthanum in heart cell culture. Effect on calcium exchange correlated with its localization. J. Cell. Biol., 54, 441.

Langer, G.A., Frank, J.S. and Tellisch, J.H. (1974). Coupling calcium in mammalian myocardium: its source and control. Adv. Cardiol., 12, 162. Karger Press, Basle.

Mommaerts, W.F.H.M. (1974). Chemical energy and cardiac work. Adv. Cardiol., 12, 116. Karger Press, Basle.

Martonosi, A. (1972). Biochemical and clinical aspects of sarcoplasmic reticulum function. In "Current Topics in Membranes and Transport". eds. Bronner and Kleingeller, 3, 83. Academic Press, London.

McNutt, N.S. and Fawcett, D.W. (1969). The ultrastructure of the cat myocardium. Atrial muscle. J. Cell. Biol., 42, 46.

Nayler, W.G. (1966). Influx and efflux of calcium in the physiology of muscle contraction. J. Clin. Orthop. Rel. Res., 46, 157.

Nayler, W.G. (1973). An effect of ouabain on the superficially-located stores of calcium in cardiac muscle cells. J. Mol. Cell. Cardiol., 5, 101.

Nayler, W.G. (1975). The plasma membrane and sarcoplasmic reticulum of muscle. In Mammalian Cell Membranes". Eds. G.A. Jamieson and D.M. Robinson. In Press.

Nayler, W.G. and Merrillees, N.C.R. (1964). Some observations on the fine structure and metabolic activity of normal and glycerinated ventricular muscle of toad. J. Cell. Biol., 22, 533.

Nayler, W.G. and Merrillees, N.C.R. (1971). Cellular exchange of calcium. In "Calcium and the Heart" p.24. Eds. Harris and Opie. Academic Press, London.

Nayler, W.G. and Dunnett, J. (1974). Regulation of myocardial contraction. In Adv. Cardiol., 12, 45. Karger Press, Basle.

Perry, S.V. (1975). In "Contraction and Relaxation in the Myocardium" Chapter 2. Ed. Nayler. Academic Press, London.

Schwartz, A. (1971). Calcium and the sarcoplasmic reticulum. In "Calcium and the Heart". Eds. Harris and Opie. Academic Press, London.

Schwartz, A., Lindenmayer, G.E. and Allen, J.C. (1972). The Na^+,K^+-ATPase membrane transport system. Importance of cellular function. In "Current Topics in Membranes and Transport". Eds. Bronner and Kleingeller. Vol. 3. Academic Press, London.

Simpson, F.O., Rayns, D.G. and Ledingham, J.M. (1974). Fine structure of mammalian myocardial cells. In Adv. Cardiol., 12, 15. (Karger Press, Basle).

Sommer, J.R. and Johnson, E.A. (1970). Comparative ultrastructure of cardiac cell membrane specializations. Am. J. Cardiol., 25, 184.

Peachey, L.D. (1965). The sarcoplasmic reticulum and transverse tubules of frog's sartorius. J. Cell. Biol., 25, 209.

Reuter, H. and Beeler, G.W. (1969). Calcium current and activation of contraction in ventricular myocardial fibers. Science, 163, 399.

Weber, A. (1966). Energized calcium transport and relaxing factors. Current Topics Bioenerg., 1, 203.

Weber, A., Herz, R. and Reiss, I. (1964). The regulation of myofibrillar activity by calcium. Proc. Roy. Soc., 3, 160, 489.

Wood, E.H., Heppner, R.L. and Weidmann, S. (1969). Inotropic effects of electric currents. Circ. Res., 24, 209.

The Contractile and Regulatory Proteins of the Myocardium

S. V. PERRY

Department of Biochemistry, University of Birmingham, U.K.

The biochemical processes occurring in muscle can be conveniently classified into three main aspects, namely those associated with the contractile, the energy-producing and the regulatory systems respectively (Fig. 1). Differences between the various types of muscle largely reside in the relative degrees of development and biochemical activity associated with these three systems.

As the main tissue for utilization of ATP in the body muscle has a highly developed system of ATP production but different types of muscle cell differ in their relative dependence on anaerobic and aerobic pathways for production of this triphosphate. For example, whereas fast skeletal muscle is highly dependent on ATP production by the glycolytic

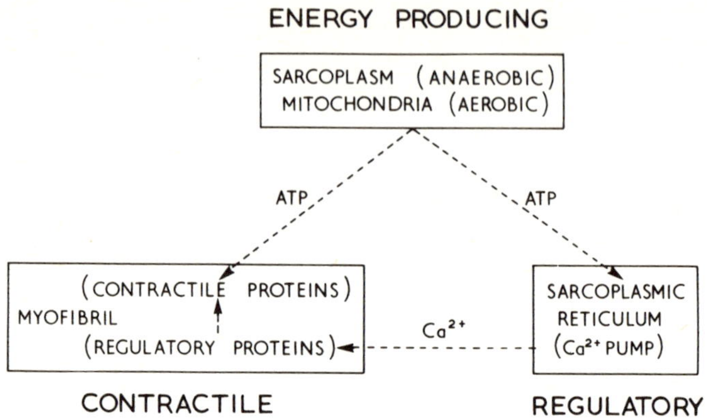

Fig. 1 The biochemical activity of striated muscle. Diagram representing the intracellular localisation of the main biochemical processes occurring in muscle and their interrelationships.

pathway, the more efficient oxidative phosphorylation is the main source of ATP in the myocardial cell with its high mitochondrial content. The systems used for energy production in muscle are widely distributed in all tissues. On the other hand the contractile and regulatory systems are highly specialized in muscle and dominate the structure of the cell in that they can, in fast skeletal muscle, for example, constitute up to 70% of the total protein present. Nevertheless, even proteins of the type associated with the latter systems may not be unique to muscle for recent research indicates that proteins very similar to those associated with contraction and regulation are widely distributed in other tissues, although in much smaller amounts than in muscle (Pollard and Weihing, 1974).

The structure of the contractile system localized in the myofibril is relatively constant in all types of mammalian striated muscle and few, if any, structural features which are unique to cardiac muscle have been observed by electron microscopic study (Simpson et al., 1973). The regulatory system, however, which consists of at least three components, namely the cell membrane, the sarcoplasmic reticulum and the regulatory proteins of the myofibril, shows much more variation between muscle types. In cardiac muscle the differences in gross structure are confined to the extra-myofibrillar components of the regulatory system, the membrane and sarcoplasmic reticulum. These aspects will be described elsewhere in this volume (Chapter 1).

In this article the protein components of the cardiac myofibril will be discussed in relation to the sequence of events that occurs when the Ca^{2+} concentration of the sarcoplasmic increases from the diastolic level of 10^{-7} M to 10^{-5} M at systole.

Detailed knowledge of the cardiac myofibril is very much less advanced than that of the myofibril of fast skeletal muscle upon which most of the studies have been made. Practically all the information has been derived from work carried out in experimental animals and very little work has been carried out on the myofribillar proteins of human skeletal or cardiac muscles. The work on experimental animals indicates in general that the results obtained from skeletal muscle can be extrapolated to cardiac tissue. Nevertheless, despite the apparent similarity in structure of the myofibril, as revealed by the electron microscope, clear differences at the primary and quaternary levels of structure are apparent in the individual proteins of the myofibril from cardiac and skeletal muscle (see Table 1).

ORGANIZATION OF PROTEINS IN THE MYOFIBRIL

The organization of the contractile and regulatory proteins in the A and I filaments is understood with some precision so far as skeletal muscle is concerned (Fig. 2). In the latter tissue according to Morimoto and Harrington (1973; 1974) myosin constitutes 96.5% of the A filament and the C protein (Offer, 1972) is the only other protein present in significant amounts. The characteristic repeat of 143Å associated with the A filament that is observed in X-ray diffraction studies corresponds to the cross bridges of about 120 Å in length that are considered to represent the head regions of the myosin molecules. In their original model Huxley and Brown (1967) proposed that the projections corresponding to the heads of the myosin molecules which gave rise to the cross bridges were arranged in a two-stranded 6/1 helix. Thus according to this model two cross bridges would occur every 143Å (Fig. 3). Although it has not always been concluded that each cross bridge

Table 1 THE PROTEINS OF THE MYOFIBRIL

Contractile		Structural
Myosin *	Tropomyosin *	α-Actinin
Actin	Troponin complex: Inhibitory protein, Troponin I *	β-Actinin
	Calcium sensitizing protein, Troponin C *	Fibrillin
	Troponin T *	M line Protein
		Z line Protein
		C Protein
70%	10-15%	10-15%

* Structural differences in cardiac muscle

projection on the A filament corresponds to the head of one myosin molecule, such a relationship would on general grounds seem to be the

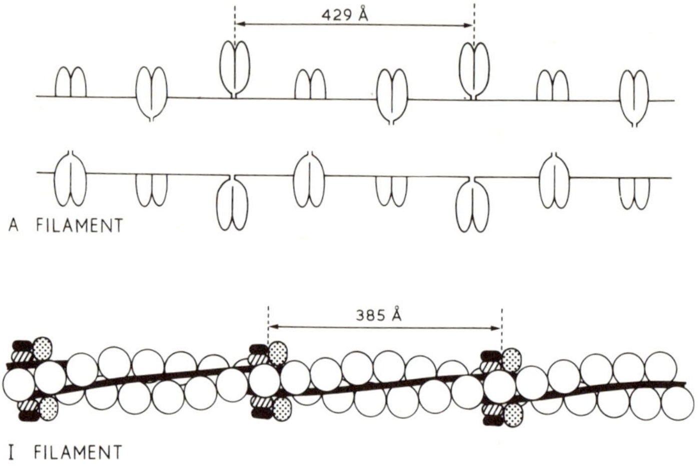

Fig. 2 Diagrammatic representation of the A and I filaments of the myofibril from skeletal muscle. In this diagram the cross bridges consisting of the two heads of the myosin molecule are represented as proposed by Huxley and Brown (1967), i.e. in a 2-stranded 6/1 helix. It is possible that the correct arrangement is the three-stranded 9/1 helix discussed by Squire (1973). See text and Fig. 3. The troponin complex is assumed to consist of one molecule each of troponin C (black), troponin I (cross-hatched) and troponin T (stippled). The tropomyosin (dark line) is represented as lying in each groove of the actin filament.

most probable. If this is the case some difficulties arise with the two-stranded 6/1 helix model. In 1963 Huxley pointed out that a considerable discrepancy existed between the number of cross bridges he could estimate from electron micrographs and the number of myosin molecules presumed to be present in the A filament. More recent direct determinations give values in the range of 3-4 myosin molecules per 143Å of A filament. Probably the most likely arrangement is the three-stranded 9/1 helix arrangement of Squire (1973) which would give three cross bridges each consisting of the head region of a myosin molecule per 143Å (Fig. 3).

There is less ambiguity about the fine structure of the I filament which is built up from two filaments composed of linearly arranged actin monomers arranged to form a helix containing 13 monomers per turn of 770Å. The repeat distance corresponding to the cross over of the two actin chains is 385Å and gives rise to a characteristic reflection on the meridian in X-ray diffraction studies. In each of the two grooves of the actin filament is localized a tropomyosin filament formed from the linear aggregation of tropomyosin molecules. Thus both actin and tropomyosin extend along the length of the I filament. On the other hand the molecule of the troponin complex which consists of one molecule each of troponin C, troponin I and troponin T is arranged at intervals of 385Å, i.e. one for every seven actin monomers. The evidence for a periodic distribution of the troponin complex along the I filament in fast skeletal muscle is now

	(a)	(b)	(c)
No. of strands	2	3	4
Residues per turn	6	9	12
Pitch (nm)	86·4	129·6	86·4
	HUXLEY & BROWN (1967)	SQUIRE (1971, 1972)	

Fig. 3 Possible arrangements of the cross bridges on the A filament. The diagrams represent cross sections through the A filament at the points where the cross bridges, consisting of the heads of the myosin molecules, project, i.e. every 14.3 nm;
(a) is the structure originally proposed by Huxley and Brown (1967) and is incorporated in Fig. 2;
(b) probably fits the evidence available better but requires to be substantiated by direct evidence.

strong. Electron microscope studies on the addition of whole troponin complex and the components derived from it to actin filaments indicate that they are responsible for the bands of electron dense material observed every 400Å, a localization first suggested by studies of the distribution of the ferritin-labelled antibody to the troponin complex (Ohtsuki et al., 1967). This conclusion has also been confirmed by X-ray diffraction studies of glycerated fibres treated with antibody to troponin C (Rome et al., 1973). In these preparations the meridional reflection corresponding to the actin 385Å repeat is enhanced 3-5 times on addition of the antibody indicating a distribution of troponin C along the I filament with this periodicity. This result correlates well with the direct estimation of the amount of troponin C present by an isotope dilution technique (Head and Perry, 1974) which indicates that one molecule of troponin C is present for 7 actin monomers. Similar X-ray data is not yet available for troponin I and troponin T but *in situ* these proteins would be presumed to be associated with troponin C and the evidence from skeletal muscle at least indicates, that each is present in an equimolar ratio in the troponin complex. In the case of rabbit heart muscle the isotope dilution method indicates that troponin C is present in a slightly lower weight per gram wet weight of muscle than is the case in fast skeletal muscle, but the content is similar to that present in slow skeletal muscle. If the myofibril content of the myocardium is taken as 45%, this corresponds to a molar ratio of troponin C to actin monomer of 1:7 (Head and Perry, 1974). Thus despite the shortage of data obtained directly on heart, the evidence implies that the relationship of actin to troponin C (and probably to the whole troponin complex) is the same in cardiac as in skeletal muscle.

MECHANISM OF CONTRACTION

It is now generally accepted that contraction takes place by relative movement between the I and A filament systems (Huxley, 1969). For contraction alone only the proteins actin and myosin are required, provided adequate concentrations of ATP and Mg^{2+} are present and the ionic conditions are such to ensure that the proteins exist as filamentous aggregates rather than in free solution. Contraction of such systems can be demonstrated with model systems, for example by super-precipitation of suspensions of actomyosin prepared from pure actin and myosin from skeletal muscle. Also with actomyosin suspensions it can be demonstrated that Ca^{2+} is not essential for contraction which will occur when Mg^{2+} only is present providing that the ionic conditions are such that the substrate $MgATP^{2-}$ is hydrolysed at a significant rate. In the myofibril where, in addition to the contractile proteins, the protein components of the regulatory system are present, Ca^{2+} is essential for $MgATP^{2-}$ hydrolysis and contraction.

Although the precise details of the mechanism which results in the relative movement of the A and I filaments is not yet fully understood, a plausible hypothesis has been evolved which draws on the evidence from X-ray, electron microscope, transient state kinetic and other biochemical investigations. Movement is presumed to occur by repeated sequences of a cyclical process which probably involves a number of stages. Each complete cycle results in relative movement of 5-10 nm and the system is restored to a state from which the cycle can be repeated. The scheme which incorporates ideas from a number of investigators, e.g. Huxley, 1969; Lymm and Taylor (1971; see Taylor, 1972) is illustrated in Fig. 4 (i) - 4(iv).

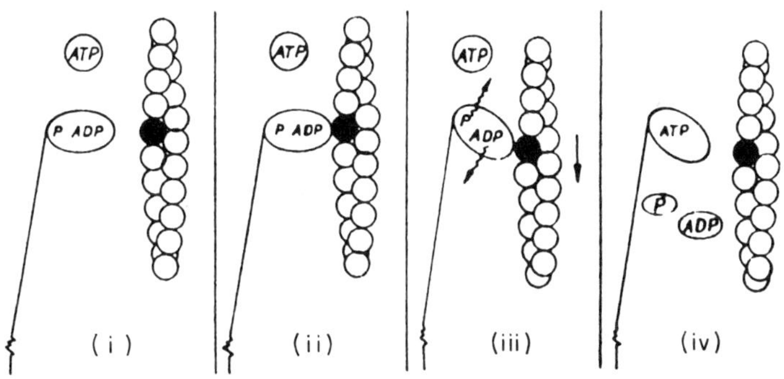

Fig. 4 Scheme to represent changes that occur in the myosin head region and at the actin filament during the hydrolysis of one molecule of ATP. In this scheme no attempt is made to illustrate the role of the regulatory protein system of the myofibril which is not shown in the diagram. The transformation, whilst attached to actin, of myosin in the conformation represented in stages (i) and (ii) to that represented in (iii) and (iv) releases mechanical work. The hydrolysis of ATP is thought to occur between stages (iv) and (i). See text for further details. (from Mannherz et al., 1973).

(i) Resting stage, diastole. The two filament systems are not linked by cross bridges. The active centres of the myosin heads are charged with the enzyme-products complex. In this form the ATP is bound to the enzyme as inorganic phosphate and ADP, the release of which products is the limiting stage of hydrolysis of ATP. This process is very slow and therefore the rate of hydrolysis of ATP is very slow.

(ii) Excitation. As a result of excitation Ca^{2+} is released into the sarcoplasm and the concentration rises to $\gg 10^{-5}$M. Troponin C binds Ca^{2+} and changes are initiated in the whole troponin-tropomyosin system that permit actin monomers to interact with the myosin heads. A cross bridge between the two filament systems is thus formed.

(iii) Contraction, systole. The interaction of actin and myosin followed by the loss of inorganic phosphate and ATP involves, in a way not precisely understood, a conformational change in the myosin molecule. As a result of the conformational change that takes place it can be postulated a change in the angle between the myosin head and the actin monomer occurs at the site of interaction. The actin monomer would then be expected to move in the direction indicated to a thermodynamically more favourable position, possibly maintaining a similar relative geometry between the sites of interaction on the actin and myosin. Thus in effect the actin is accelerating the hydrolysis of ATP by speeding the release of products from the myosin, the rate limiting step in ATP hydrolysis, and at the same time moving in relation to the myosin molecule due to the changes in conformation of the myosin head region.

(iv) Relaxation. When the products are released from the active site of myosin a new ATP molecule combines with myosin, the interaction with actin is broken and the ATP bound to the myosin is rapidly converted into the enzyme products complex (see stage (i)). At the same time the myosin returns to the conformation characteristic of resting muscle and is ready to undergo a further cycle providing the Ca^{2+} concentration is high enough to enable the regulatory system to permit interaction to occur once again.

The above series of events is triggered off by a rise in the free Ca^{2+} concentration to about 10^{-5}M, whilst the Mg^{2+} and ATP concentrations remain essentially constant. It can be deduced from the information in Table 2 that both in resting and in contracting muscle virtually all the ATP present will be in the $MgATP^{2-}$ form. Myosin alone hydrolyses ATP at a rate comparable to that occurring during contraction only in the presence of concentrations of Ca^{2+} which are much higher than ever occurs *in vivo*. Under these circumstances, $CaATP^{2-}$ is the substrate and is hydrolysed rapidly. On the other hand the hydrolysis of ATP in the presence of Mg^{2+} is very slow for $MgATP^{2-}$ is a poor substrate for myosin alone (Fig. 5). In this property myosin behaves rather differently from most other enzymes that have ATP as a substrate, which usually work well

Table 2 ADENOSINE TRIPHOSPHATE AND DIVALENT CATION CONCENTRATIONS IN RESTING AND CONTRACTED MUSCLE

	Resting	Contracted
ATP (mM)	3-8	3-8
Mg (mM)	8-15	8-15
Ca (mM)	1×10^{-4}	1×10^{-2}
ATPase activity	Low	High
Actin-myosin bonds	Broken	Formed

in the presence of Mg^{2+}. In the presence of actin under conditions which the latter protein can interact with myosin, however, $MgATP^{2-}$ is split rapidly and under optimum conditions the rates are comparable to those obtained _in vivo_ during contraction in mu:cle. Thus the control of contractile activity is essentially a problem of enzyme regulation which depends on the rather unique properties of myosin ATPase.

The mechanism of this effect of actin on the enzymic activity of myosin is not understood but it follows that activity is regulated in muscle by controlling the interaction of actin with myosin and hence the rate of ATP hydrolysis and the concomittant conformational changes which lead to contraction. Despite the adequate levels in resting muscle, ATP is

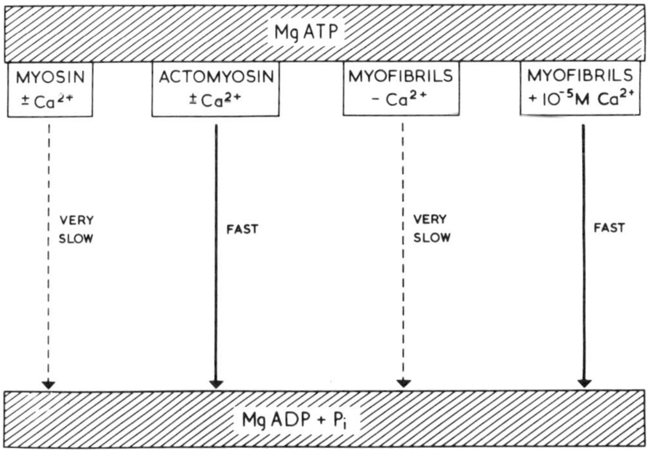

Fig. 5. Scheme summarizing the effect of Ca^{2+} on the hydrolysis of $MgATP^{2-}$ by myosin, actomyosin and myofibrils. The scheme indicates the rates of ATP hydrolysis by the various systems under conditions similar to those applying in the muscle cell, i.e. Mg^{2+} and ATP concentration in the millimolar range and Ca^{2+} in the range 10^{-7} - 10^{-5}M. Under these conditions virtually all of the ATP will be in the form $MgATP^{2-}$.

not split at any significant rate in the resting phase because the enzyme is in effect myosin alone.

It should be noted that although the Ca^{2+} concentration increases about one hundred times during excitation, even at its highest concentration it is still only about one hundredth of that of the Mg^{2+}. Nevertheless such is the power of discrimination of troponin C for Ca^{2+} that even in the presence of 5-10 mM Mg^{2+} and decimolar K^{+}, Ca^{2+} is selectively bound by the protein and brings about changes in the regulatory protein system which permit interaction of actin and myosin to initiate the contractile cycle (Perry, 1974).

REGULATORY PROTEIN SYSTEM

The regulatory protein system of muscle consists of tropomyosin and the troponin complex and has the function of conferring Ca^{2+} sensitivity on the hydrolysis of $MgATP^{2-}$ by the actomyosin system. Its effect is illustrated in Fig. 6 which compares the effect of the EGTA (ethanedioxybis (ethylamine) tetra-acetate), a high specific chelating agent for Ca^{2+}, on the Mg^{2+}-stimulated ATPase of actomyosin composed of actin and myosin freed from regulatory proteins and on the myofibril. In the former system removal of traces of Ca^{2+} by EGTA has no effect on the ATPase activity and the slight inhibitory effects at higher EGTA concentration are due to chelation of a significant fraction of the Mg^{2+} present. With myofibrils, however, very low concentrations of EGTA, 1% or less of the concentration of Mg^{2+} brings about sharp inhibition of the ATPase activity. This is due to removal of traces of Ca^{2+} present in the system and which are essential for a high rate of the Mg^{2+}-stimulated ATPase of the myofibril (Perry and Grey, 1956a; 1956b). This

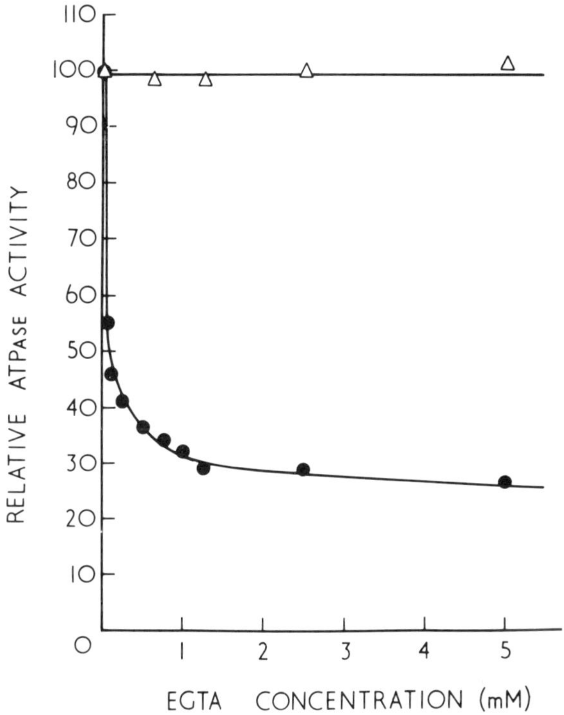

Fig. 6 Ca^{2+} sensitivity of the Mg^{2+}-stimulated ATPase of myofibrils and desensitized actomyosin. ATPase assays carried out in 2.5 mM ATP, 2.5 mM $MgCl_2$ and 25 mM tris-HCl buffer)pH 7.6) at 25°C.

Δ Desensitized rabbit actomyosin (Schaub et al., 1967).

● Rabbit myofibrils.

effect lead to the discovery by Ebashi and collaborators (Ebashi and Kodama, 1965; Ebashi et al., 1969) that tropomyosin and a not previously recognised protein, troponin, now known to consist of three components of different function, are both essential for Ca^{2+} regulation of the ATPase activity of the myofibril. Although the precise mechanism of the system cannot yet be described, fractionation of the complex and investigation of these properties of the components, have given some insight into the processes involved. The three components of the troponin complex, whose properties are listed below, are considered to be present in equimolar proportions in skeletal muscle and probably also in cardiac muscle, although there is no direct information as to relative amounts of the components present in the latter tissue.

Troponin C. This component is the target protein for calcium and undergoes conformational changes when 2 Ca^{2+} are bound per molecule. There is some disagreement on the number of binding sites for Ca^{2+} per mole of troponin C from skeletal muscle. Values reported in the literature vary from two to four with the high affinity sites possessing a stability constant in the range $10^6 - 10^7 M$. Although it has no effect itself in the Mg^{2+}-stimulated ATPase of actomyosin, troponin C neutralises the inhibitory action of troponin I on this enzymic system.

Troponin I. Troponin I is a highly specific inhibitor of the Mg^{2+}-stimulated ATPase of actomyosin. It does not inhibit the Ca^{2+}-stimulated ATPase and therefore its function is in some way to prevent the effect of actin in activating the hydrolysis of $MgATP^{2-}$ by myosin. The inhibitory effect is much accentuated by tropomyosin, the specific activity in the case of troponin-I from fast skeletal being increased three to four times in the presence of this protein. Troponin C neutralises the inhibitory activity of troponin I both in the absence and presence of Ca^{2+}. Troponin I also forms a complex with troponin C that is stable to 8M urea when Ca^{2+} is present.

Troponin T. Although it is present in all troponin preparations the biological activity of troponin T is not so clearly defined as in the case of the other two components. It forms a complex with tropomyosin and is essential for complete reconstitution of Ca^{2+} sensitivity when the troponin components are recombined.

The function of the troponin complex is summarized in Fig. 7 where the effects of various combinations of components of the regulatory protein system on the Mg^{2+}-stimulated ATPase of actomyosin in the presence and absence of Ca^{2+} are illustrated. It should be noted that although tropomyosin is essential for calcium sensitivity of the Mg^{2+}-stimulated ATPase, a partial restoration of sensitivity of the actomyosin ATPase Ca^{2+} can be demonstrated when the whole complex is replaced by troponin I and troponin C. For complete reconstitution of the Ca^{2+} sensitivity troponin T is required in addition to the other three components (Perry *et al.*, 1972).

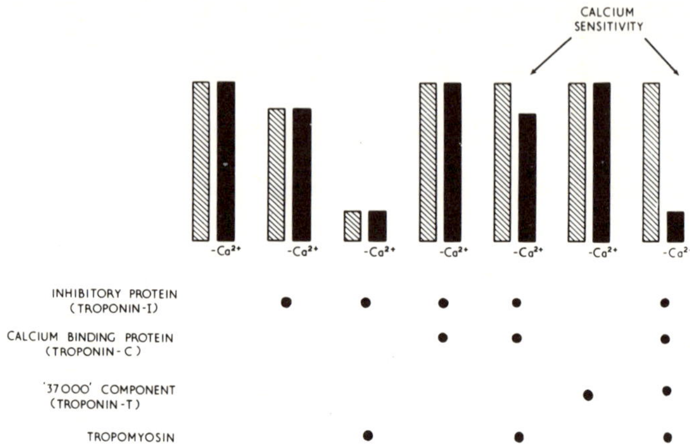

Fig. 7 Schematic representation of the effects of various combinations of the components of the regulatory system of skeletal muscle on the Mg^{2+}-stimulated ATPase of actomyosin in the presence of Ca^{2+} and EGTA. ATPase activity of actomyosin measured in 25 mM Tris-HCl (pH 7.6), 2.5 mM $MgCl_2$, 2.5 mM ATP with 0.1 mM $CaCl_2$ present (hatched histograms) and 2 mM EGTA (blocked histograms). The components added to the system are represented by black dots beneath the pairs of histograms. From Perry (1974).

SPECIAL FEATURES OF THE CONTRACTILE AND REGULATORY PROTEINS FROM CARDIAC MUSCLE

Actin

Of all the proteins under discussion actin appears to be the most consistent in structure in different types of muscle. In rabbit fast skeletal muscle it consists of a single polypeptide chain of 374 amino acid residues folded into a globular possibly somewhat ellipsoid molecule of diameter 55Å and molecular weight 42000 (Table 3). All actins analysed so far contain one residue per mole of the unusual amino acid, 3-methyl histidine. As yet there have been no reports of differences between actin from skeletal and cardiac actins (Katz and Carstens, 1963; Katz and Maxwell, 1964; see Katz, 1970). These studies have failed to distinguish any significant differences in amino acid composition, physical properties or in size and shape in cardiac actin. The studies so far carried out, however, would not have detected minor differences in sequence such as conservative amino acid replacements. The primary sequence of actin from rabbit fast muscle is now known (Elzinga et al., 1973) and the final decision as to whether actin of skeletal and cardiac muscle are identical must await primary sequence studies on the latter protein. The relative constancy of the actin structure would imply that its role is such that it is little affected by the different physiological properties of the various types of muscle cell.

Myosin

Of the proteins under discussion myosin was probably the first that was shown to exhibit differences from its skeletal counterpart. Over thirty years ago Bailey (1942) reported that the ATPase activity of cardiac

Table 3. MOLECULAR WEIGHTS AND QUATERNARY STRUCTURE OF MYOFIBRILLAR PROTEINS FROM CARDIAC AND SKELETAL MUSCLE OF THE RABBIT

	Muscle	Mol. wt.	Quaternary Structure
Actin	Fast skeletal	42,000	Single polypeptide chain
	Cardiac	42,000	Single polypeptide chain
Myosin	Fast skeletal	4.8×10^5	2 chains of 200,000; 2 of 19,000; 1 of 22,000; 1 of 15,000
	Cardiac	4.8×10^5	2 chains of 200,000; 2 of 19,000; 2 of 24,000
Tropomyosin	Fast skeletal	68,000	α-subunit of 34,000; β subunit of 34,000
	Cardiac	68,000	2 α-subunits of 34,000
Troponin C	Fast skeletal	18,000 *	Single polypeptide chain
	Cardiac	18,000	Single polypeptide chain
Troponin 1	Fast skeletal	21,000 *	Single polypeptide chain
	Cardiac	28,000	Single polypeptide chain
Troponin T	Fast skeletal	37,000	Single polypeptide chain
	Cardiac	41,000	Single polypeptide chain

* Mol. wt. determinations from sequence analysis. Other troponin components from sodium dodecyl sulphate electrophoresis.

myosin was lower than that of skeletal myosin. Data on cardiac myosin obtained by hydrodynamic and electron microscope studies indicate that the size and shape of the molecule are very similar to myosin from skeletal muscle. Nevertheless clear differences in structure at the primary and quaternary levels exist (see Katz, 1970, for review).

The primary structural differences are not sufficiently great to be apparent from the amino acid composition of the whole molecule except in the case of 3-methyl histidine which residue is absent in cardiac myosin whereas in the protein from fast skeletal muscle there are about 1.7 residues per mole. Less 3-methyl histidine is present in myosin from slow skeletal muscle and this residue is absent from foetal skeletal muscle myosin, the heavy chain of which is not identical to that of cardiac myosin (Trayer *et al.*, 1968; Kuehl and Adelstein, 1970).

One of the most profound differences in myosin from cardiac tissue compared to that present in skeletal muscle is in its quaternary structure as revealed by polyacrylamide gel electrophoresis under dissociating conditions as, for example, in sodium dodecyl sulphate. These differences are summarized in Fig. 8. On electrophoresis in sodium dodecyl sulphate in these conditions all myosins migrate as a heavy chain fraction, molecular weight about 200,000, and a light chain fraction which is characteristic of the muscle from which the myosin is isolated. The resolution on sodium dodecyl sulphate is not good enough to show differences in the heavy

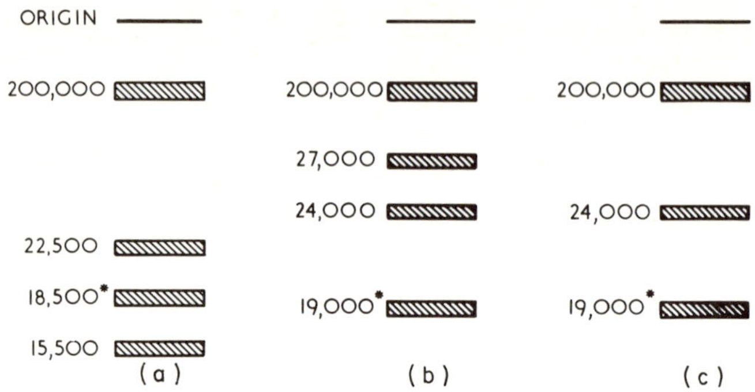

Fig. 8 The light chain components of myosin isolated from different types of striated muscle of the rabbit. Diagrammatic representation of the electropherograms obtained when myosin is electrophoresed on 10% polyacrylamide gel at pH 7.0 in the presence of 0.1% sodium dodecyl sulphate (see Perrie _et al._, 1973). The hatched areas represent protein bands stained with Coomassie Blue corresponding to the molecular weights indicated. The band marked with an asterisk is phosphorylated by myosin light chain kinase (Pires _et al._, 1974).

(a) Longissimus dorsi, psoas

(b) Soleus, crureus

(c) Heart

chains although primary structural differences undoubtedly occur in the heavy chains of fast skeletal and cardiac myosins. For example, the peptide sequence of thirteen residues, the histidine of which is methylated in skeletal myosin, has different residues in four places in cardiac myosin (Huszar, 1972). Some early work (Stracher, 1965) also suggested differences in the polypeptide sequences about the cysteine residues but in this study it was not then recognized that the light as well as the heavy chains contain different thiol sequences and the differences reported may in part be due to light chain differences.

Differences in the light chains are much better documented. Whereas the myosin from rabbit fast skeletal muscle contains three different species of light chain, cardiac myosin has only two which are not identical with those of fast skeletal muscle and probably not with those of myosin from slow skeletal muscle (Perrie, Thomas and Perry, 1973). A possible arrangement of the light chain components in the myosin molecule is suggested in Fig. 9. In both fast skeletal and cardiac muscle myosin there are four light chains for every two heavy chains and whereas cardiac myosin is apparently much more homogeneous in possessing two different light chains, fast skeletal muscle myosin has three. If it is assumed that the two globular head regions of the myosin molecule are identical, the data is best explained by assuming that there are two species of molecule present in skeletal myosin (Fig. 9).

Although obviously the two light chains of cardiac myosin are not identical with any of the skeletal myosin light chains, presumably

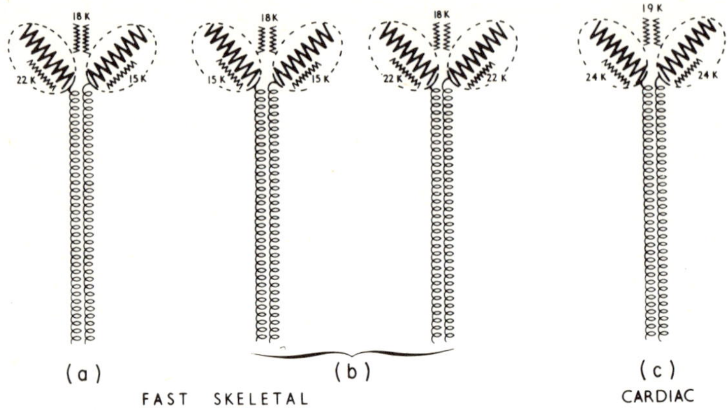

Fig. 9 Schematic representation of the structure of myosin from fast skeletal and cardiac muscles. In diagram (a) the four light chain molecules composed of three different chains are shown to be all present in one molecule. In this case the two globular head regions would not be identical but the protein would consist of one molecular species. In (b) the myosin is considered to be composed of two different molecular species with identical head regions. As cardiac muscle contains only two light chains in roughly equal proportions its structure is probably as indicated in (c). The 18,000 (18K) and 19,000 (19K) dalton light chain components are represented outside the globular heads as there is evidence from skeletal muscle that part at least of these components can be removed without loss of enzymic activity.

they have a similar function and genetic origin. The 24,000 dalton light chain of cardiac muscle has part of its amino acid sequence identical with that of the 22,000 dalton light chain of fast skeletal myosin but in addition it also contains thiol sequences that are absent from the latter (Weeds and Frank, 1972). The 19,000 dalton light chain is phosphorylated by myosin light chain kinase and is presumably similar in function to the 18,500 dalton light chain of fast skeletal myosin (Perrie, Smillie and Perry, 1973; Frearson and Perry, unpublished results).

Thus, although complete primary structural studies are not yet available, the evidence available indicates that differences exist between cardiac and skeletal myosins, both in the light and heavy chain fractions. It is not therefore surprising that cardiac myosin has a lower specific ATPase activity (Bailey, 1942; Gergely, 1959), is more resistant to tryptic digestion (Brahms and Kay, 1963; Mueller et al., 1964) and shows differences in immunological properties (see Hirabayashi and Hayashi, 1972, for review). Of the properties listed, the enzymic activity most obviously correlates with physiological function. The specific ATPase activity is about one half to one third of that of myosin from fast skeletal muscle, which is what might be expected in view of the correlation between specific ATPase activity of myosin and muscle speed (Barany, 1967).

Tropomyosin

The tropomyosin molecule consists of two polypeptide subunits of approximately equal size that form a dimer of molecular weight 68,000 (Table 3). Each polypeptide chain exists in the α-helical form and the two subunits are arranged so that a supercoil is produced by lateral association of the two chains (Crick, 1953; Cohen and Holmes, 1963; Sodek *et al.*, 1972). In this way is produced a rod-like molecule of dimension 40.0 x 2.5 nm that is able to aggregate to form fibrous network structures and paracrystals with characteristic periodicities (Woods, 1967; Cohen and Longley, 1966; Hilburn *et al.*, 1974). In the I filament such end to end aggregation of the molecules gives rise to the tropomyosin filaments which are localized in each of the two grooves of the actin filament.

Cardiac tropomyosin is the only type of tropomyosin from striated muscle which has to date shown to be homogeneous with regard to subunit structure. Tropomyosin isolated from skeletal muscle consists of two main forms of subunit, the α and β subunits. These subunits appear to have slightly different molecular weights when determined by polyacrylamide electrophoresis in sodium dodedcyl sulphate. Nevertheless, paracrystals made from purified α and β subunits show identical periodicities indicating that the molecules of α_2 and β_2 tropomyosin at least have identical packing behaviour. The most striking difference is the presence of 2 cysteine residues per mole in the β subunit compared to one in the α subunit. Cardiac tropomyosin contains only one type of subunit identical with α tropomyosin so far as can be judged from its amino composition, electrophoretic mobility, para-crystal structure and immunological properties (Cummins and Perry, 1973; 1974, Hilburn *et al.*, 1974). The relative proportion of α to β subunits varies from 3.8:1 in rabbit psoas to 1.1:1 in the soleus muscle from the same species. In general the slower the skeletal muscle the higher the proportion of β subunit present. α-Tropomyosins from skeletal muscles of different species and cardiac tropomyosins from different species cross react and are immunologically very similar, if not identical (Cummins and Perry, 1974) (Fig. 10). β-Tropomyosin appears to be species specific and rabbit antibody to it will not react with tropomyosin from striated muscle of other species. Thus the subunit of tropomyosin of cardiac muscle appears to be identical with the main tropomyosin subunit present in fast striated muscle. Unlike cardiac myosin which in certain properties resembles myosin from slow skeletal muscle, cardiac tropomyosin is more like the major tropomyosin component in fast skeletal muscle.

Troponin C

The first claim that cardiac troponin C differed from its skeletal counterpart was due to the report that the relative affinities for calcium

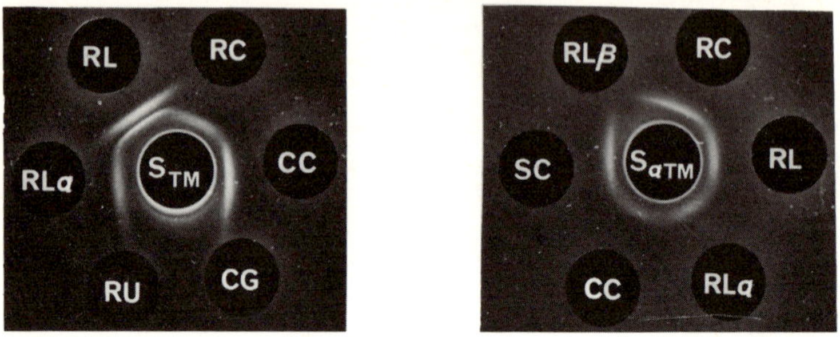

Fig. 10 Reactions of guinea pig antisera raised against tropomyosin of rabbit skeletal muscle with tropomyosins from cardiac and skeletal muscles. Aliquots (50 μl) of antigen or antisera were added to wells. Antigen solutions were in the range of 40-60 μg of tropomyosin/ml. RL, RLα and RLβ represent unfractionated, α- and β-tropomyosins of rabbit longissimus dorsi muscle respectively. S_{TM} and $S_{\alpha TM}$ represent guinea pig antisera raised against unfractionated and α-tropomyosin of rabbit longissimus dorsi muscle respectively.

(a) Reactions of tropomyosin from different muscle types with antiserum raised against unfractionated tropomyosin. RC, rabbit cardiac; CC, chicken cardiac; CG, chicken gizzard; RU, rabbit uterus.

(b) Reactions of antiserum raised against α-tropomyosin from rabbit longissimus dorsi with tropomyosins from and strontium were different (Ebashi et al., 1969). As yet there has been no published confirmation of this finding but differences in the affinities for divalent cations are likely, for clear differences in primary structure of troponin C from cardiac and skeletal muscles of the same species can be demonstrated (Hirabayashi and Perry, 1974; Head and Perry, unpublished results). This can be deduced from the amino acid compositions (Table 4), the nature of the peptides obtained on cyanogen bromide digestion and the electrophoretic mobilities of the protein under various conditions. The same criteria suggest on the other hand that troponin C of fast and slow skeletal muscle are identical (Head and Perry, unpublished results). In view of the primary structural differences it is perhaps not surprising that antibody raised against skeletal muscle from troponin C of the rabbit will react with skeletal muscle troponin C from other species but not with rabbit cardiac troponin C (Hirabayashi and Perry, 1974) (Fig. 11).

Unlike the two other components of the troponin complex with which molecular weight differences occur between the variants found in different muscle types, troponin C from skeletal and cardiac muscles

---

skeletal and cardiac muscle.

RC, rabbit cardiac; CC, chicken cardiac; SC, sheep cardiac. (From Cummins and Perry, 1974).

Table 4. AMINO ACID COMPOSITIONS OF TROPONIN COMPONENTS FROM FAST SKELETAL AND CARDIAC MUSCLES

	TROPONIN C (chicken) *		TROPONIN I (rabbit) +		TROPONIN T (rabbit)+	
	Fast Skeletal (Res/18,000)	Cardiac (Res/18,000)	Fast Skeletal (Res/21,000)	Cardiac (Res/26,000)	Fast Skeletal (Res/37,000)	Cardiac (Res/41,000)
Asp	24.9	24.6	15	20.1	24.5	33.3
Thr	6.6	7.6	3	11.5	7.1	9.6
Ser	5.8	4.9	10	13.7	10.9	11.5
Glu	30.6	30.2	33	33.9	67.6	85.0
Pro	0.9	3.5	5	9.7	11.3	14.7
Gly	12.1	12.9	8	15.1	9.4	17.3
Ala	12.2	7.8	14	24.6	29.2	28.9
Val	5.4	7.9	7	9.5	10.3	11.8
Met	9.8	9.3	9	4.0	5.2	4.5
Ile	10.1	8.1	5	8.3	10.0	13.3
Leu	9.6	12.5	17	22.7	23.4	25.2
Tyr	0	2.9	2	4.4	5.1	5.8
Phe	11.1	8.3	3	5.5	5.8	7.9

His	1.0	0.7	4	3.2	7.4	4.5
Lys	11.0	13.1	24	25.3	53.4	44.9
Arg	5.8	4.2	16	20.7	29.8	33.2
Cys	-	-	3	-	0	0
Trp	-	-	1	-	2.1	-

* From Hirabayashi & Perry 1974

\+ Unpublished results, J.M. Wilkinson, H. Syska, R. Grand & S.V. Perry

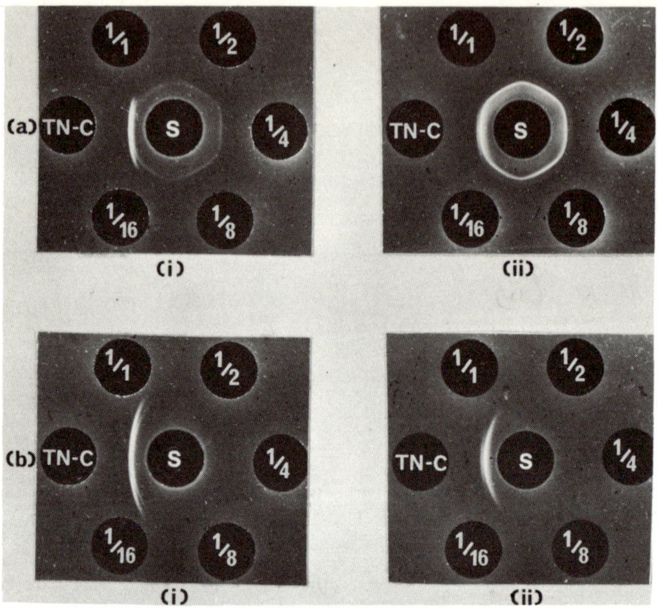

Fig. 11 Reactions of extracts of myofibrils from chicken skeletal and cardiac muscles with antiserum to chicken skeletal muscle troponin C. Anti-chicken skeletal troponin C raised in the rabbit and myofibrillar extracts prepared as described by Hirabayashi and Perry (1974). TN-C, chicken skeletal muscle 62 μg/ml; S, anti-chicken skeletal muscle troponin C. Myofibrillar extracts diluted as indicated in wells. (From Hirabayashi and Perry, 1974).

(a) Chicken skeletal myofibrillar extract in outer wells.

(i) no additions, (ii) 2 mM EGTA.

(b) Chicken cardiac myofibrillar extract in outer wells.

(i) no additions, (ii) 2 mM EGTA.

have a very similar molecular weight. Troponin C interacts with troponin I to form a stable complex in the presence of Ca^{2+} and 8M urea, which when formed between the components from cardiac muscle has a different electrophoretic mobility to that obtained with skeletal muscle (Syska *et al.*, 1974). The complex is neither tissue nor species specific and can be utilized to form a convenient affinity chromatographic method for the rapid isolation of troponin I and troponin C from whole muscle (Syska *et al.*, 1974; Head and Perry, unpublished results).

Thus, the form of troponin C found in cardiac muscle is unique to this tissue and would therefore be unlikely to possess precisely the same affinity for Ca^{2+} and other divalent cations as skeletal troponin C. The functional reasons for these differences are not clear but presumably relate to the special nature of the regulatory system of the cardiac myofibril. The differences in structure are probably not, as is the case with myosin, related to muscle speed for troponin C is apparently identical in fast and slow skeletal muscles. The amount of troponin C present in cardiac muscle is the same as a percentage of total myofibrillar protein as in skeletal muscle (Head and Perry, 1974).

Troponin I

To date three forms of this protein have been identified in striated muscle (Syska *et al.*, 1974). In the rabbit the main troponin I component of fast skeletal muscles such as longissimus dorsi and psoas differs from that of slow skeletal muscles such as the soleus or crureus. Both proteins have an apparent molecular weight of 23,000 as determined by polyacrylamide electrophoresis in sodium dodecyl sulphate but give different peptides when treated with cyanogen bromide. Also the mobilities of the complexes formed by the two forms of troponin I with troponin C from rabbit fast skeletal muscle are different. From amino acid sequence analysis the true molecular weight of troponin I from rabbit fast skeletal muscle is 21,000 (Wilkinson and Grand, 1974).

Troponin I of cardiac muscle has a higher apparent molecular weight of 28,000 when estimated by electrophoresis in sodium dodecyl sulphate. The amino acid analysis is clearly different from that of fast skeletal troponin I (Table 4). The mobility of the complex with fast skeletal troponin C is similar to that obtained with slow skeletal muscle troponin I. Limited studies on the biological activity of cardiac troponin I isolated by affinity chromatography indicate that it is less effective as an inhibitor of the Mg^{2+}-stimulated ATPase than troponin I from fast skeletal muscle when both are tested with desensitized actomyosin from fast skeletal muscle (Syska _et al._, 1974; Syska and Perry, unpublished results). The significance of this is not clear yet; a possibility which is currently under investigation is that it may be related to the extent of phosphorylation of cardiac troponin I (See below).

Troponin T

The role of troponin T is less well understood than those of the other components of the complex and it is therefore difficult to decide on the significance of differences which exist in this component from different muscle cell types. The data so far available is not as precise as in the case of the other components of the troponin complex but there are strong suggestions that, as is the case with troponin I, different forms of troponin T exist for fast skeletal, slow skeletal and cardiac muscles. It is also similar to troponin I, but unlike the other myofibrillar proteins, in that the apparent molecular weight of troponin T as determined by electrophoresis in sodium dodecyl sulphate varies according to the muscle type from which it is isolated. There does not appear to be a consistent trend for whereas troponin T of fast rabbit white muscle has a molecular weight of 37,000, that of chicken breast muscle is about 44,000 and that of the slower chicken leg muscle is 37,000. Rabbit cardiac troponin T has an apparent molecular weight of about 41,000 and the complement of peptides obtained on digestion with cyanogen bromide shows some differences to those obtained from troponin T of fast skeletal muscle (Jackson and Perry, unpublished observations).

PHOSPHORYLATION OF MYOFIBRILLAR PROTEINS

There is little doubt that changes in Ca^{2+} concentration of the sarcoplasm is the major factor in regulating contractile activity in striated muscle in general and in cardiac tissue in particular. Nevertheless, it is unlikely that a simple mechanism involving the troponin system as outlined above is the only mode of regulating contractile activity in muscle. The regulation of biochemical processes tends to be complex and usually involves several interlocking processes. Muscle, whether it be of the cardiac or skeletal type, is unlikely to be unique in this respect.

Regulation of the biological activity of proteins by phosphorylation is now well established as a phenomenon (Holzer, 1973; Huijing and Lee, 1973) and the recent demonstrations that the light chains of myosin (Perris _et al._, 1972; 1973) and troponin (Stull _et al._, 1972; Pratje and Heilmeyer, 1972; Perry and Cole, 1973; 1974) undergo phosphorylation and dephosphorylation by enzymes present in muscle raises the question of the significance of these mechanisms for muscle function.

Myosin Phosphorylation

The enzyme myosin light chain kinase (Pires _et al._, 1974) specifically phosphorylates the light chain of 18,000-19,000 of myosin that is present in myosin isolated from fast and slow skeletal and cardiac muscle (see Fig. 8). Indeed a light chain of the size that can be phosphorylated is the most consistent feature of the light chain fraction of different types of myosin. As yet most of the information on phosphorylation has been obtained with both myosin and the light chain kinase isolated from fast skeletal muscle. In the latter system one serine residue in a unique sequence (Perris *et al.*, 1973) is phosphorylated by the light chain kinase and is readily dephosphorylated by an enzyme present in sarcoplasm and associated in small amounts with purified myosin preparations. Myosin light chain kinase requires Ca^{2+} for activity and the enzyme will therefore be active during contraction and probably not during relaxation. The significance of this fact is not yet understood but implies that if phosphorylation occurs it can only take place during the excitation stage. As yet there is no direct evidence that phosphorylation followed by dephosphorylation occurs during the contractile cycle *in vivo*. The presence in muscle of a specific kinase for the process, however, implies that the system has functional significance.

Although the role of light chain phosphorylation is not yet clear the process appears to be a general property of myosins. The light chain kinase from fast skeletal muscle phosphorylates the 19,000 light chains of slow skeletal and cardiac muscle, although the rate of the process with the latter as substrate is about 50% of that obtained with the appropriate light chains of myosin from fast and slow skeletal muscle. Myosin light chain kinase can be isolated from cardiac muscle and there are preliminary suggestions that it may not be identical with the enzyme isolated from fast skeletal muscle (Frearson and Perry, unpublished).

Troponin Phosphorylation

The initial reports of phosphorylation of troponin relate to the complex isolated from skeletal muscle (Bailey and Villar-Palasi, 1971; Stull *et al.*, 1972; Pratje and Heilmeyer, 1972; Perry and Cole, 1973). It is now clear that troponin from rabbit fast skeletal muscle prepared by the standard procedures involving isolation of the whole complex (see Perry and Cole, 1973; 1974) contains approximately one molecule of covalently bound phosphate per mole, almost all of which is on troponin T (Perry and Cole, 1973; 1974). On phosphorylation of the whole complex with ATP and phosphorylase kinase from rabbit skeletal muscle the phosphate content can be increased up to about three moles per mole, most of this being incorporated in Troponin T and 20% or less of the additional phosphate being incorporated in troponin I. Cyclic AMP-dependent protein kinase from bovine cardiac muscle slowly phosphorylates the troponin complex, in this case practically all of the phosphate going on to troponin I. As yet there has been no evidence of phosphorylation of troponin C.

Cardiac troponin shows some differences to the skeletal protein in that when isolated by the standard procedures it contains quite large amounts of 3'5'-cyclic AMP-dependent kinase (Reddy *et al.*, 1973;

Perry and Cole, 1974) so that on addition of ATP under the appropriate ionic conditions it is phosphorylated at a high rate which is not significantly increased by addition of a bovine cardiac muscle 3'5'-cyclic AMP-dependent kinase. The rate of phosphorylation is five to ten times faster than is obtained with the bovine protein kinase on troponin from fast skeletal muscle, which has no endogenous protein kinase activity when isolated (S.V. Perry and H.A. Cole, unpublished results).

The endogenous 3'5'-cyclic AMP-dependent kinase or the added bovine cardiac enzyme selectively phosphorylate troponin I. If troponin I is isolated by affinity chromatography directly from fresh muscle the protein from fast skeletal muscle contains about 1 mole phosphate/mole whereas the cardiac protein isolated under the same conditions contains 1-3 moles of phosphate/mole protein.

Thus there is good evidence that troponin I exists *in situ* as the phosphorylated form and in cardiac muscle at least one of these sites is readily phosphorylated by a 3'5'-cyclic AMP-dependent kinase present in the muscle. Enzymes are present in cardiac muscle to dephosphorylate these sites for phosphate is readily lost from troponin I during isolation. It is too early to say whether phsophorylation of cardiac troponin I is of any significance in modifying the contractile response. Nevertheless this is the first demonstration of a myofibrillar protein that can be phosphorylated at a substantial rate by a 3'5'-cyclic AMP-dependent protein kinase. It is tempting to suggest that this phenomenon is concerned in the inotropic effect of the catecholamines. Such a hypothesis has some attraction for the changes stimulated by 3'5'-cyclic AMP could lead to modification of protein-protein interactions. The process involves adding several negative charges to troponin I which normally has a small net positive charge at physiological pH values and which plays a central role in regulating ATPase activity by modulating the interaction between actin and myosin.

CONCLUSIONS

It is clear that the myofibrillar system in cardiac muscle is essentially identical with that in skeletal muscle in gross structural features. Nevertheless, with the exception of actin, all the proteins of the contracto-regulatory system that have been studied in detail show differences at the primary level of structure. The differences are not simple substitutions of amino acid residues but often involve significant differences in amino acid composition and in molecular weight, e.g. myosin light chains, troponin I and troponin T. Quite apart from the precise nature of these structural differences, our understanding of the mechanism of contraction and its regulation at the myofibrillar level is not yet great enough to enable us to understand the functional significance of these special features of the cardiac myofibrillar proteins. The obvious conclusion would be that they have been selected out by evolutionary processes for a special role in the contractile activity of cardiac muscle. It is unlikely, however, that they are responsible for any major differences in the mechanism of contraction and its regulation in cardiac muscle compared to skeletal muscle. They are probably involved in modulation of the general mechanism to accommodate the special features of cardiac muscle function.

The uniqueness of most of the cardiac myofibrillar proteins suggests that certain of them, for example, troponin C or troponin I, could be of special significance for the immunopathology of this tissue. For example, the detection of cardiac troponin C in serum might provide a highly specific index of myocardial cell damage.

The rapid advance of knowledge of the primary structure of the myofibrillar proteins as demonstrated by the elucidation of the amino acid sequences for actin, troponin I, troponin C and tropomyosin during the past few years implies that the myofibril, or at least the I filament, will soon be described with a three-dimensional detail unique for an organelle. Such advances made with skeletal muscle proteins cannot fail to have a similar impact on the understanding of the cardiac system. Thus the cardiologist will be in a unique position to understand the major functional part of the cardiac cell in molecular terms.

This knowledge of the myofibrillar system should lead the way to the development of new pharmacological agents. Up to now the pharmacology of muscle has depended largely on drugs which exert their effect on the membrane of the cell and trigger a series of intracellular events ultimately leading to changes in the enzymic of the myofibril. The new knowledge could point the way to the design of drugs with greater precision of activity, for example, acting directly on the contracto-regulatory system of the myofibril. Advances such as this would contribute considerably to the pharmacology of muscle in general and heart in particular.

REFERENCES

Bailey, C. & Villar-Palasi, C. (1971) Fed. Proc. 30, 1147.

Bailey, K. (1942) Biochem. J. 36, 121-139

Barany, M. (1967) The Contractile Process, 197-216. Supplement to J. Gen. Physiol. 50

Brahms, J. & Kay, C.M. (1963) J. Biol.Chem. 238, 198-205

Cohen, C. & Holmes, K.C. (1963) J. Mol.Biol. 423-432

Cohen, C. & Longley W. (1966) Science, 152, 794-796

Crick, F.H.C. (1953) Acta Crystallogr. 6, 689-697

Cummins, P. & Perry, S.V. (1973) Biochem. J. 133, 765-777

Cummins, P. & Perry, S.V. (1974) Biochem. J. 141, 43-49

Ebashi, S., Endo, M. & Ohtsuki, I. (1969) Quart.Rev. Biophys. 2, 351-384

Ebashi, S. & Kodama, A. (1965) J. Biochem. 58, 107-108

Elzinga, M., Collins, J.H., Kuehl, W.M. & Adelstein, R.S. (1973) Proc.Nat.Acad.Sci. USA, 70, 2687-2691.

Gergely, J. (1959) Ann. N.Y. Acad.Sci. 72, 538-554

Head, J.F. & Perry, S.V. (1974) Biochem. J. 137, 145-154

Hilburn, M.E., Cummins, P. & Perry, S.V. (1974) J.Mol.Biol. in the press

Hirabayashi, T. & Hayashi, Y. (1972) Development, Growth and Differentiation, 14, 133-165

Hirabayashi, T. & Perry, S.V. (1974) Biochem.Biophys.Acta. 351, 273-289

Holzer, H. (1973) Symp.Soc.Expl.Biol. 37, 319-331

Huijing, F. & Lee, E.Y.C. (1973) Protein Phosphorylation in Control Mechanisms. Academic Press, London and New York.

Huszar, G. (1972) Nature New Biol. 240, 260-264

Huxley, H.E. (1963) J. Mol. Biol. 7, 281

Huxley, H.E. (1969) Sci. 164, 1356-1366

Huxley, H.E. & Brown, W. (1967) J. Mol. Biol. 30, 383-434

Katz, A.M. (1970) Physiol.Rev. 50, 63-158

Katz, A.M. & Carstens, M.E. (1963) Circulation Research 13, 474-479

Katz, A.M. & Maxwell, J.B. (1964) Circulation Research 14, 345-350

Kuehl, W.M. & Adelstein, R.S. (1970) Biochem. Biophys.Res.Com. 39, 956-964

Lymn, R.W. & Taylor, E.W. (1971) Biochemistry 10, 4617-4624

Mannherz, H.G., Leigh, J. Barrington, Holmes, K.C. & Rosenbaum, G. (1973) Nature New Biol. 241, 226-229

Morimoto, K. & Harrington, W.F. (1973) J. Mol. Biol. 77, 165-175

Morimoto, K. & Harrington, W.F. (1974) J. Mol.Biol. 83, 83-97

Mueller, H., Theiner, M. & Olson, R.E. (1964) J. Biol.Chem. 239, 2153-2159

Offer, G. (1972) Cold Spring Harbor Symp. Quant. Biol. 37, 87-95

Ohtsuki, I., Masaki, T., Nonomura, Y. & Evashi, S. (1967) J. Biochem. (Tokyo) 61, 817-819

Perrie, W.T., Smillie, L.B. & Perry, S.V. (1972) Cold Spring Harbor Quant. Biol. 37, 17-18

Perrie, W.T., Smillie, L.B. & Perry, S.V. (1973) Biochem. J. 135, 151-164

Perrie, W.T., Thomas, M.A.W. & Perry, S.V. (1973) Biochem.Soc. Trans. 1, 860-861

Perry, S.V. (1974) Biochem.Soc.Symp. 39, 115-132

Perry, S.V. & Cole, H.A. (1973) Biochem. J. 131, 425-428

Perry, S.V. & Cole, H.A. (1974) Biochem. J. in the press

Perry, S.V. & Grey, T.C. (1956a) Biochem. J. 64, 184-192

Perry, S.V. & Grey, T.C. (1956b) Biochem. J. 64, 184, 5P

Perry, S.V., Cole, H.A., Head, J.F. & Wilson, F.J. (1972) Cold Spring Harbor Symp. Quant. Biol. 37, 251-262

Pires, E., Perry, S.V. & Thomas, M.A.W. (1974) FEBS Lett. 41, 292-296

Pollard, T.D. & Weihing, R.R. (1974) CRC Critical Reviews of Biochem. 2, 1-68

Pratje, E. & Heilmeyer, L.M.G. (1972) FEBS Lett. 27, 89-93

Reddy, Y.S., Ballard, D., Giri, N.Y. & Schwartz, A. (1973), J.Mol.Cell.Cardiology, 5, 461-471

Rome, E., Hirabayashi, T. & Perry, S.V. (1973) Nature New Biol. 244, 154-155

Schaub, M.C., Hartshorne, D.J. & Perry, S.V. (1967) Biochem.J. 104, 263-269

Simpson, F.O., Rayns, D.G. & Ledingham, J.M. (1973) In Ultrastructure of the Mammalian Heart, p.1-41, Ed. by C.E. Challice & S. Viragh, Academic Press, New York & London

Sodek, J., Hodges, R.S., Smillie, L.B. & Jurasek, L. (1972) Proc. Nat.Acad.Sci. USA, 69, 3800-3804

Squire, J.M. (1971) Nature 233, 457-462

Squire, J.M. (1972) J. Mol.Biol. 72, 125-138

Squire, J.M. (1973) J.Mol.Biol. 77, 291-323

Stracher, A. (1965) In Muscle, Proceedings of Symp. held at the Faculty of Medicine University of Alberta (1964) Edited by W.M. Paul, E.E. Daniel, C.M. Kay & G. Monckton, p.85-92 Pergamon Press Ltd.

Stull, J.T., Brostrom, C.O. & Krebs, E.G. (1972) J. Biol.Chem. 247, 5272-5274

Syska, H., Perry, S.V. & Trayer, I.P. (1974) FEBS Lett. 40, 253-257

Taylor, E.W. (1972) Ann.Rev.Biochem. 41, 577-616

Trayer, I.P., Harris, C.I. & Perry, S.V. (1968) Nature(Lond) 217,452-453

Weeds, A.G. & Frank, G. (1972) Cold Spring Harbor Symp. on Quant. Biol. 37, 9-14

Wilkinson, J.M. & Grand, R.J.A. (1974) In the press

Woods, E.F. (1967) J.Biol.Chem. 242, 2859-2871

Cardiac Contraction

M. I. M. NOBLE and G. H. POLLACK

Midhurst Medical Research Institute, Sussex, U.K.
and Departments of Anesthesia and Bioengineering,
University of Washington, U.S.A.

INTRODUCTION

In previous chapters the anatomical arrangement of structures within the myocardial cell have been described. It seems clear that the contractile function of the cell is finally subserved by interactions between filaments composed of contractile proteins. The other components of the cell are primarily concerned with the delivery of energy in the form of high energy phosphate and the control of contraction and

*Dr. Pollack is an Established Investigator of the American Heart Association.

relaxation. We will assume in this chapter that this control is achieved via activator calcium ion, the intracellular concentration of which rises to bring on contraction and falls to produce relaxation. The evidence for this crucial role of the calcium ion is briefly reviewed by Ebashi (1972), from whom further references may be obtained. In this chapter we will discuss the possible mechanisms by which interaction can take place between filaments of contractile protein in order to produce force and movement. Then we will apply these mechanisms to try to interpret some of the major elements of cardiac mechanics.

MECHANISMS OF CONTRACTION

Structural Basis

There now appears to be a wide measure of agreement that the thick and thin filaments slide relative to one another rather than contract or buckle. We do not propose to review all the evidence presented in the past for and against these two viewpoints. The crucial evidence in favour of the sliding filament hypothesis is that the width of the A-band remains constant, regardless of sarcomere length. All the length changes take place within the I-band (A.F. Huxley, and Niedergerke, 1954 ; H.E. Huxley, and Hanson, 1954). This is illustrated in Figure 1 which presents a schematic diagram of a sarcomere with an adjacent half sarcomere on its right. Electron micro-

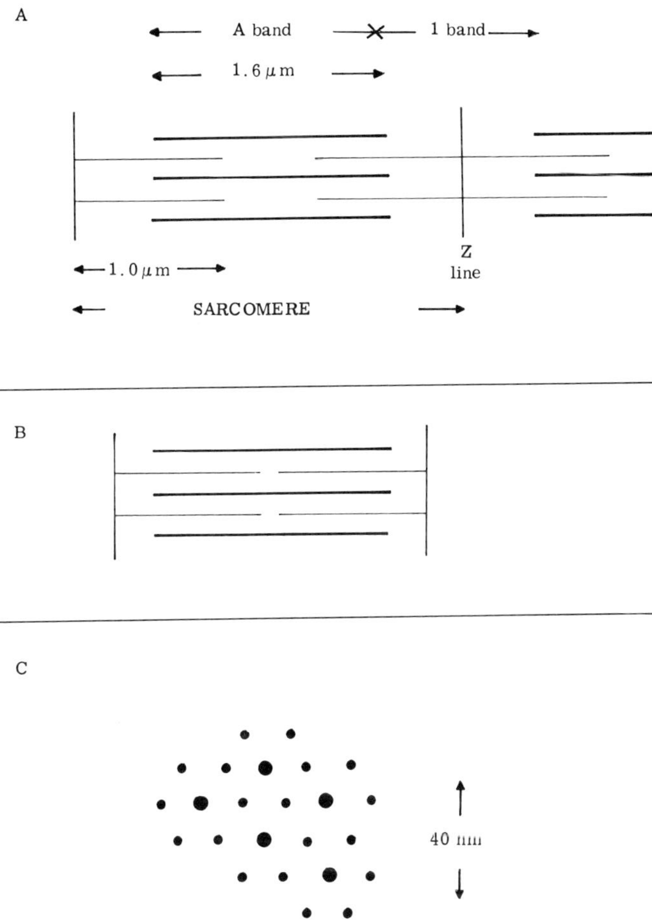

Figure 1

graphic evidence suggests that within the A-band there is a parallel array of thick filaments composed predominantly of myosin. From each Z line at the ends of the sarcomere thin filaments composed of actin and other proteins extend towards the centre of the sarcomere, and interdigitate with the thick filaments. Two different sarcomere lengths are depicted in panels A and B of the figure, to illustrate the way in which the A-band remains at a constant length. The only conclusion to be drawn from this type of anatomical evidence is that the sarcomeres shorten due to a movement of the thin filaments toward the centre of the sarcomere, sliding between the thick filaments. The implication is that during the change from rest to activity the contractile proteins comprising these filaments interact in such a way that a force is generated tending to pull the thin filaments inward.

Any mechanism proposed to explain the generation of such a force must take into account the arrangement of the filaments in the third dimension, which is illustrated in panel C of the figure; this is a schematic cross-section of a sarcomere in the area of thick and thin filament overlap, and shows that the thin filaments are disposed around the thick filaments in hexagonal arrays (although such disposition differs in certain species).

More recently, information has emerged about the finer structure of these filaments (see previous chapters) ; of these newer features the greatest importance has been attached to the lateral projections from the thick filaments which extend in the direction of the thin filaments. These often can be seen in electron micrographs. Their dynamics are inferred from the results of X-ray diffraction studies. These have indicated a transfer of mass during activation from the thick to the thin filament (Miller and Tregear, 1970) which seems to indicate that these projections, or cross-bridges, attach to the thin filaments during activation, and therefore are likely to be involved with the generation of force.

The Cross-Bridge Theory

Out of these structural elements have arisen the cross-bridge theories (A.F. Huxley, 1957 ; Davies, 1963 ; H.E. Huxley, 1969 ; A.F. Huxley and Simmons, 1971). Their essential feature is that there is a physical link formed between the projections on the thick filaments and the thin filaments, and that force is generated through these links. These ideas are summarized in Figure 2 which represents perhaps the most detailed exposition of the cross-bridge theory (H.E. Huxley, 1969 ; A.F. Huxley and Simmons, 1971). The theory assumes that there are active sites on the thin filament at regular intervals along its length and that during sliding the cross-bridges interact with these sites. In each interaction the head of the myosin molecule rotates, thus stretching the connecting link (AB in Figure 2); it is this stretched link, AB, which transmits the force between thick and thin filament. The instantaneous force depends upon the instantaneous number of stretched links. If the muscle is not constrained to constant length, then the rotation of these

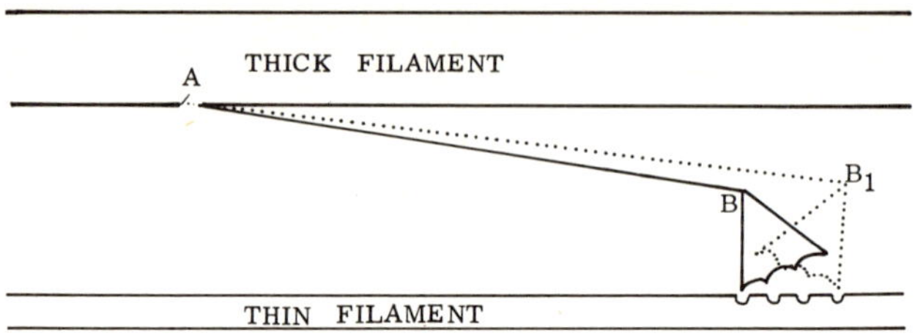

Figure 2

heads will cause the thin filaments to be displaced with respect to the thick filaments (leftward in Figure 2) and the sarcomere will shorten.

It is fair to say that the essence of this theory, although perhaps not all details, is widely viewed as adequate to explain most data. It fits well with electron micrographic and X-ray diffraction results, and has been shown to be consistent with many mechanical properties of muscle, although not necessarily all (Julian, 1971). There is one important area, however, where the cross-bridge theory may prove to be inadequate: stability. By stability we mean the following: Given the known structure of muscle, and assuming contraction occurs according to the cross-bridge theory, could the muscle maintain structural integrity during contraction, or would the filament lattice break apart, or collapse? This neglected area deserves some thought.

(a) Longitudinal Stability

A striking feature of the electron micrographs of skeletal and

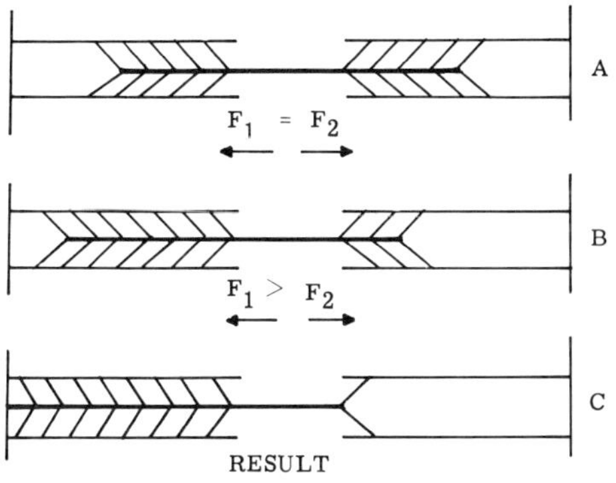

Figure 3

cardiac muscle available to us in the literature is the constancy with which the myosin filaments are found to be centrally placed within the sarcomere during relaxation and contraction (Figure 1). This indicates that the force acting between the two sets of filaments is generated in such a way that this stable equilibrium position is maintained. Does the cross-bridge theory lead to such stability? Consider Figure 3. In panel A is illustrated a thick filament with two of its surrounding six thin filaments on either side. During activity a number of cross-bridges would be formed and force would be generated on the left half of the thick filaments with one set of thin filaments and on the right half with another set of thin filaments. If the number of cross-bridges in the two halves of the sarcomere is the same, the force generated on each half of the thick filament will be the same and the thick filament will remain in a central position. However, during activity it is likely that peturbations would occur, such as that illustrated in panel B, so that the number of cross-bridges on one half of the sarcomere might transiently exceed the number of the other half. This would result in a difference in force on the two halves of the thick filament, tending to further increase this unbalance. Since no restoring forces have been postulated in the cross-bridge theory, the result would be as shown in panel C, i.e. the thick filament would be pulled over to one or the other Z-line, which does not seem to happen in reality. Thus the assumption of the cross-bridge mechanism gives rise to longitudinal instability.

Another manifestation of longitudinal instability is illustrated in Figure 4. The isometric force-sarcomere length relation, after Gordon, Huxley, and Julian (1966), is shown at the top. The two points on the curve represent hypothetical sarcomeres in series having slightly different initial lengths. The diagram below illustrates the degree of overlap of thick and thin filaments for each of the two sarcomeres. The one at the left can develop more force because there are more cross-bridges available than in the one on the right. Therefore, during isometric contraction, the sarcomere at the left will shorten and stretch the one at the right; the more this occurs, the greater the unbalance and the more it will continue to occur. This instability will

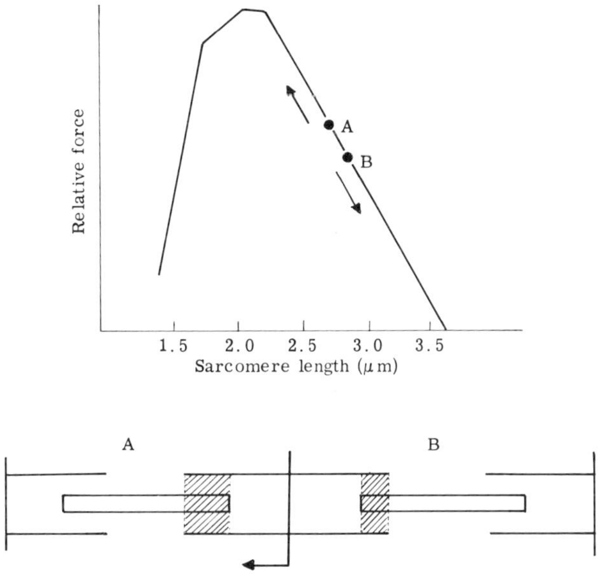

Figure 4 Top. Length-force curve of muscle.

Below. Adjacent sarcomeres A & B with lengths equal to points A & B on the length-force curve above. Cross-hatched area indicates area of filament overlap.

give rise to two populations of sarcomere lengths growing further and further apart, a situation which does not occur in reality (Cleworth and Edman, 1972).

It seems evident from the two examples presented above that if longitudinal stability is to be achieved with the cross-bridge mechanism (as it must), a more complex mechanism than has been proposed to date needs to be postulated.

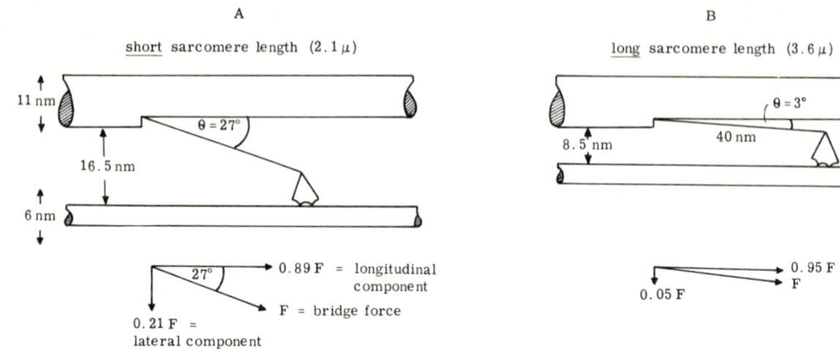

Figure 5 The longitudinal and lateral components of the cross-bridge force generated in the model of H.E. Huxley and A.F. Huxley and Simmons

(b) Lateral Stability

Another striking feature of electron micrographs of muscle is the stable arrangement of the lattice as seen in cross-section (Figure 1-C). X-ray diffraction data indicate not only that this lattice structure is preserved during force generation, but that the spacing does not change appreciably from rest to activation (Elliott, Lowy, and Millman, 1967). Is the cross-bridge theory consistent with preservation of the lattice?

An attached cross-bridge is shown in Figure 5A. When force is developed the link AB pulls on the thick filament. But the force is not only in the longitudinal direction. As shown in the lower portion of Figure 5A, it is applied obliquely, so that there is also a lateral component of cross-bridge force. In the absence of an equal and opposite lateral force between thick and thin filaments the result would be aggregation of all the filaments into a core in the centre of the cross-section of the sarcomere. In other words this mechanism gives rise to marked lateral instability. In order that lateral stability be achieved an additional mechanism producing a repulsive force between thick and thin filaments which is equal and opposite to the lateral component of cross-bridge force must be postulated.

This equal and apposite force could not be a simple one. First it would need to be time varying during a twitch since the number of cross-bridges, hence the sum of lateral components of cross-bridge force within the sarcomere, varies with time. Second, it must vary with sarcomere length in two different ways. First the number of cross-bridges changes, and hence the lateral component does as well. Second, X-ray diffraction data have shown that as sarcomere length in intact fibers is increased by stretch, the filaments are drawn together laterally in such a way that sarcomere volume is preserved (Elliott, et al., 1963). Therefore, when a cross-bridge attaches at longer sarcomere length the angle of attachment, θ , decreases (Figure 5B) and the lateral component force of each cross-bridge is decreased. If the lateral restoring force is to remain equal and opposite, it must somehow sense the separation of the myofilaments.

As Gale and Davies (1973) have pointed out the repulsive restoring force between myofilaments would have to be larger when the filaments are further apart laterally, a kind of force unknown in physics.

Similar questions of stability arise with earlier, simpler cross-bridge theories (A.F. Huxley, 1957). But these older versions have largely given way to the current one for many reasons, perhaps the most important of which relates to the subject just discussed, lateral filament separation. Gordon, Huxley and Julian (1966) demonstrated that developed tetanic force is related directly to the amount of overlap of thick and thin filament (at lengths above 2 μ). Interpreted in terms of the cross-bridge theory, one is led to conclude that the force is dircetly proportional to the number of activated cross-bridges, and further, that each cross-bridge generates the same force regardless of sarcomere length, hence filament separation. This would not be the case with the earlier, relatively short cross-bridge (Figure 6) since the angle θ between cross-bridge and longitudinal axis would change quite a lot with filament separation. The longitudinal component of cross-bridge force would vary accordingly. In order that a given cross-bridge develop the same longitudinal force component at differing interfilament distances, the long arm, AB, had to be postulated as in Figure 2 (H.E. Huxley, 1969). By comparing 5A and 5C, it is seen that the longitudinal component of force is not

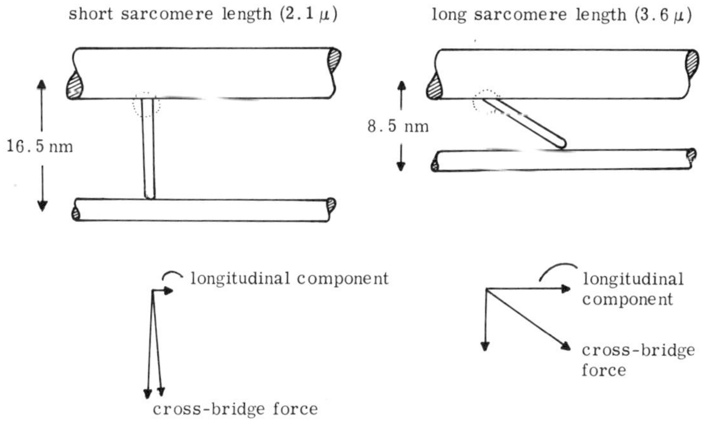

Figure 6 The dependence of the longitudinal component of the force of an individual cross-bridge on sarcomere length.

very much different for the two lateral interfilament spacings. Thus the mechanical data are satisfied by this more complex arrangement.

To summarize, it appears that the concept of muscle force generation by cross-bridges has led to the evolution of a rather complex mechanism. While this mechanism seems compatible with much ultra-structural, biochemical, and biophysical data, the question of stability has not yet been addressed seriously. To us, this seems a crucial question, as stability is a condition necessary for the existence of such a mechanism.

(c) Electrostatic Theories

Other theories offer mechanisms far different from those of cross-bridges. Most of these involve electrostatic forces among best known being those of Ingels and Thompson (1966) and Elliott et al., (1970). In the former, force is generated by a coulomb force between the negatively charged thick filament and the positively charged thin filament. This theory is subject to the same question of lateral stability as the cross-bridge mechanism . In the latter theory a lateral repulsive force is postulated to exist between filaments which results in a shortening force because of the constant volume constraint within the sarcomere. However, recent studies have shown that constant volume is not a general attribute of muscle. For instance, Elliott and Matsubara (1972) have shown that constant volume is not preserved with stretch of skinned fibers, while contraction can still occur, apparently quite normally.

Innumerable other theories have appeared, the merits or demerits of which are beyond the scope of this chapter. However, there is one theory (Iwazumi, 1970) which has received little attention, but seems to us worthy of further scrutiny. The principle of force generation is that of a dielectric rod in the field between the plates of a capacitor (Figure 7A). The dielectric rod is always sucked into the field. Iwazumi supposes that the thin filament is the dielectric rod and the cross-bridges on the thick filament generate the field (7B). It is supposed that the cross-bridges are approximately the same length as generally thought (Figure 2 and 5) but that they extend laterally, like spokes radiating from the thick filament thus they extend beyond

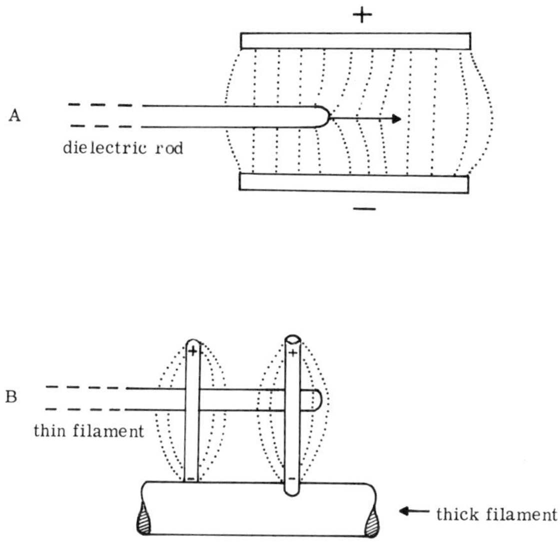

Figure 7 A. Principle of Force generation proposed by Iwazumi.

B. Suggested mode of field generation suggested by Iwazumi.

the thin filaments. Force is generated as charge is separated on the cross-bridge and an electric field built up (Figure 7B), a process which involves the presence of calcium.

This mechanism is stable, both longitudinally and laterally. Since the longitudinal force depends upon the interaction of the field and the <u>tip</u> of the thin filament rather than the entire rod, the number of activated cross-bridges does not come into play and the instability illustrated in Figure 3 does not apply. The mechanism has lateral stability because there is no significant component of lateral force generated by this mechanism.

Like the cross-bridge theory, this theory has also been demonstrated to be compatible with a wide range of ultrastructural, biochemical, and biophysical observations. For example, the length-tension curve is explained in terms of variations, with sarcomere length, of the amount of charge possibly brought about by variation in the amount of calcium around the tips of the thin filaments. The force-velocity relation and the changes of force brought about by quick-stretches or quick-releases (discussed below) are the result of voltages induced on the capacitors by thin filament movement. Thus, by virtue of its predictive ability, its simplicity, and its stability, we fell that this theory is promising and ought to be subject to further test, perhaps along the lines outlined by Iwazumi, himself. It is already possible to object to some detailed aspects of the theory e.g. the cross-bridges do not seem to project beyond the thin filaments. Cross-bridge morphology is far from certain and varies from muscle to muscle e.g. in giant barnacle fibres the cross-bridges extend from thick to thick filament throughout the A band (Hoyle et al., 1973). The morphological evidence is just as difficult to reconcile to the cross-bridge theory which requires a 40 nm long bridge projecting very obliquely in a longitudinal direction. The Iwazumi theory does not take into account the conformational changes in the contractile proteins (Perry, this book). However the principle of force generation is compatible with these findings. The theory may be restated in more general terms as follows:- During the change from rest to activity there are conformational changes in the contractile proteins associated with a separation of charge around the tips of filaments which, behaving as dielectric cylinders, are then pulled within the field (Figure 7A).

RELATION OF THEORIES TO CARDIAC MECHANICS

There are several aspects of cardiac mechanics we would like to consider to examine the extent to which these can be predicted by the molecular theories of contraction.

Series Elasticity

If a muscle is stimulated to contract, but prevented from shortening, it develops force isometrically as illustrated in Figure 8A (dashed curve). If during this time the muscle is allowed to shorten suddenly there is a rapid drop in force similar to that obtained in a recoiling spring. This has generally been explained in terms of a series elastic element (Hill, 1938 ; Jewell and Wilkie, 1958). This idea supposes that the muscle consists of a contractile element and elastic element in series, and that during isometric force development the contractile element shortens and stretches the series elastic element; when a rapid shortening step is imposed recoil takes place

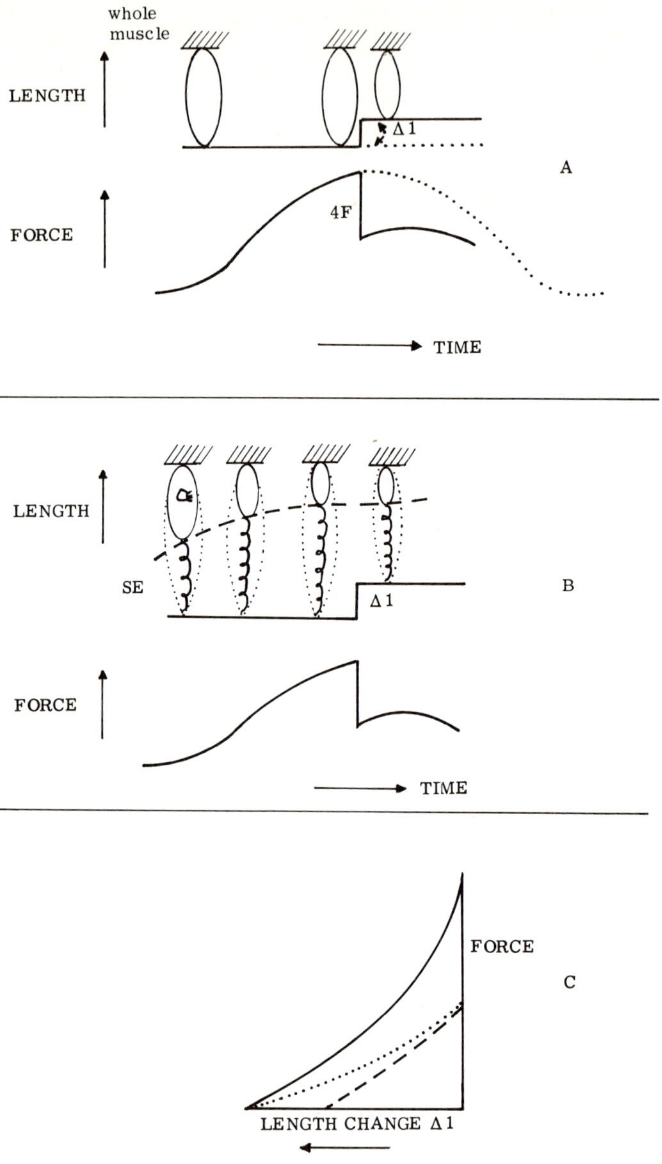
whole
muscle
LENGTH
Δ1
A
4F
FORCE
TIME
LENGTH
SE
Δ1
B
FORCE
TIME
FORCE
C
LENGTH CHANGE Δ1

Figure 8.

in the series elastic element with no change in the length of the contractile element (Figure 8B). A plot of force against the amplitude of the shortening step, ΔL, would then give the characteristics of the series elastic element (Figure 8C, solid curve). If the shortening step is imposed at an earlier time when the force generated is less, one should according to this model obtain a segment of exactly the same curve as before, starting from a lower force. This is shown by the dashed line in Figure 8C which was obtained by horizontal displacement of the solid curve to the right. The dotted line in this Figure shows how muscle actually behaves. The forces immediately after rapid shortening from the lower force are reduced by the same ratio as the reduction in the initial force. This means that if the sudden drop in force is due to the recoil of elastic structures, the number of these elastic structures must increase with the development of isometric force in proportion to that force. This is explained by A.F. Huxley and Simmons (1971) by postulating that there is a virtually instantaneous elasticity within each cross-bridge; they suggest that this compliance could reside in the link AB, Figure 2. Thus the isometric force developed depends on the number of cross-bridges formed, and the active stiffness (determined by the stiffness of the links AB) also depends upon the number of cross-bridges tormes, explaining the result obtained in Figure 8C.

The length step required to drop the force to zero in skeletal muscle is about 15 nanometers per half sarcomere, although Huxley and Simmons argue that the true value is likely to be less than this. The length of the link AB is not known, but 40 nanometers may be a reasonable estimate (H.E. Huxley, 1969). Thus an extension during isometric contraction of 15 nanometers suggests that these links would be rather compliant.

In heart muscle however, these links would have to be unreasonably compliant. The data of Noble and Else (1972) and Pollack et al., (1972) suggest that heart muscle also behaves in the manner illustrated in Figure 8C. In the case of heart muscle however, the shortening step required to drop force to zero is about 5 times as much as in skeletal muscle. This would mean an extension of the link AB during isometric contraction of approximately 75 nanometers. This would seem unreasonably high if the resting length of the link is only 40 nanometers.

Thus it appears that elasticity of cardiac muscle is not readily explained by the cross-bridge theory, alone.

In Iwazumi's theory, the phenomenon of series elasticity is explained in an entirely different way (Figure 9). As the thin filament (dielectric rod) moves into the capacitor, the effective dielectric constant between the plates increases, thereby increasing the capacitance.

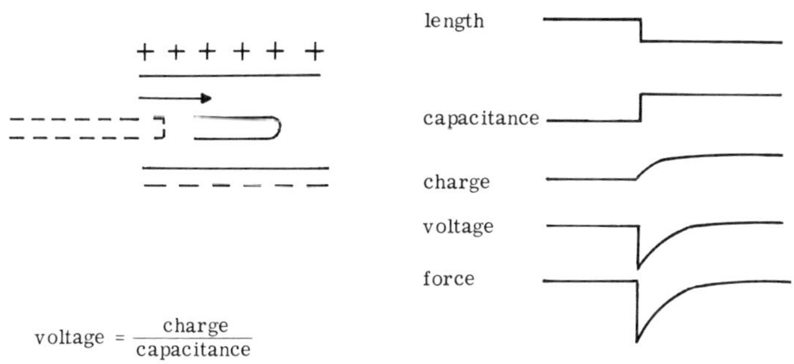

Figure 9 Quick release phenomenon according to Iwazumi's theory.

If this is done so quickly (quick release) that the charge on the capacitor has no time to leak, the voltage decreases abruptly (voltage = charge divided by capacitance) giving rise to a sudden drop of force.

Iwazumi's theory encounters similar difficulty in explaining the differences between cardiac and skeletal muscle of the magnitude of the length change needed to drop the force to zero. It would be necessary to increase the width of the field (i.e. the capacitor plate length) by a factor of five to account for the results in cardiac muscle, clearly unlikely. However, differences in the cardiac and skeletal muscle contractile proteins (Perry, this book) would lead one to expect quantitative differences in the quick release response in the two types of muscle on this basis.

The answer may lie elsewhere. To date, changes of sarcomere length during a quick release or quick stretch of cardiac muscle have not been observed. All observations have been confined to muscle length. One possibility is that for a release of say 8% muscle length required to drop the force to zero, the sarcomeres shorten by only 1-2%, similar to skeletal muscle. The remainder of the shortening could be in the damaged ends of the muscle (damaged as a consequence of mounting in clips, or tying). Recent observations using laser diffraction techniques on mammalian papillary muscle (Krueger, Christensen and Pollack, in preparation) indicate that such damaged ends are considerably stretched by contracting sarcomeres during isometric contraction; these ends might well be expected to recoil upon release, and could represent a large portion of the series compliance in cardiac muscle.

Thus the elastic properties of cardiac sarcomeres are unknown. Until the proper measurements have been carried out, it seems premature to try to apply theories of contraction, and certainly premature to conclude they are inadequate. It will be noted from Figure 9 that Iwazumi's theory predicts that with a quick release, the force drops suddenly and then immediately develops at a slower rate. This is how sarcomeres actually behave (Huxley and Simmons, 1970). In order to explain this according to cross-bridge theory one must postulate that during the redevelopment phase more cross-bridges are attaching (Podolsky and Nolan, 1973) or that a further mechanical change is taking place within a fixed number of cross-bridges, (Huxley and Simmons, 1971).

The results of Ford, Huxley and Simmons (1974) favour the latter suggestion since the behaviour indicated by the continuous line in Figure 8C is adhered to fairly closely throughout the force redevelopment period. However it is important to emphasise that these results are equally compatible with any force generating mechanism which itself produces the force changes actually seen when the sarcomere is subjected to a quick release. Such mechanisms include the Iwazumi principle (Figure 9).

The Force - Length Relation

It is well known that cardiac muscle contracts more vigorously when stretched. Traditionally, this has been explained in terms of the degree of overlap of thick and thin filaments and hence the number of cross-bridges (Leyton and Sonnenblick, 1971). At optimum length, where further stretch will no longer bring about increased force, it is thought that a maximum number of cross-bridges can be formed. However, recent studies in living mammalian heart muscle (Pollack and Huntsman, in press) indicate that the major portion of the force-length curve of heart muscle encompasses only a narrow range of sarcomere lengths, several tenths of a micron. This is a range over which the number of cross-bridges could not be expected to change dramatically simply as a result of overlap differences.

A further complication is that there appears to be a great deal of sarcomere shortening during isometric contractions of isolated cardiac muscle. This seems to be true in both frog heart (Johnson, et al., CIBA Symposium in press) and mammalian heart (Krueger, Christensen and Pollack, in preparation). It seems likely that contractions in which the sarcomeres remained truly isometric may not yet have been observed in isolated heart muscle. Until such a force-sarcomere length relation can be measured, it seems, again, premature to apply molecular theories of contraction to interpret the force-length relation of cardiac muscle.

It is quite possible that the molecular mechanism, *per se*, may not be the most relevant factor needed to explain the myocardial force-length relation. Length dependent effects on excitation-contraction coupling may be more important determinants of the ascending limit of the length force curve in both cardiac and skeletal muscle. Taylor and Rüdel (1970) and Rüdel and Taylor (1971) have presented evidence that the fall off of force in single fibers of frog skeletal muscle at short lengths (below 2.2 μ) may be related to lowered activation levels. There are some data in cardiac muscle which indicate that the level of activity may also be length dependent (Blinks, 1970 ; Nilsson, 1972).

The Force - Velocity Relation

It is well known that there is an approximately hyperbolic

relation between force and velocity in muscle (Hill, 1938). This is a consistently reported feature of skeletal muscles, but is not always found in cardiac muscle (e.g. Noble et al., 1969; Meiss and Sonnenblick, 1972). Rather the force-velocity hyperbola seems distorted in one way or another, depending upon the specific technique used to make the measurements.

The earlier version of the cross-bridge theory, (Huxley, 1957) predicted the hyperbolic force-velocity relation. This relation was based upon the concept that the higher the relative velocity of translation of the filaments, the lower the probability of cross-bridge formation, and therefore, the lower the force. The newer, more complex version of this theory (Huxley and Simmons, 1971) has not yet been demonstrated to explain, quantitatively, the force-velocity relation.

In Iwazumi's theory, the force-velocity relation is explained as follows: Each time the thin filament tip enters a capacitor during shortening, it increases its capacitance, thereby tending to decrease the voltage and field, and hence the force. The faster this occurs (the extreme being the quick release, illustrated in Figure 9) the more the force drops. The slower it occurs, the more time is available for the charge to build up on the capacitor plates so as to restore the voltage which existed before the rod entered the capacitor i.e. for the lower velocities, the voltage and therefore the force is higher. In this way the inverse relation between velocity and force is obtained.

Can these theories account for the more complex force-velocity relations found in cardiac muscle? Perhaps not if they are really found at the sarcomere level. But, measurements of the relation between force and sarcomere shortening velocity have not yet been carried out. Thus, it is unknown whether these relations are indeed as straight-forward as in skeletal muscles, or whether complicating factors such as cellular inhomogeneity and absence of tetanus in cardiac muscle might give rise to relatively more complex force-sarcomere velocity relations.

CONCLUSION

It will be apparent from this discussion that the mechanism by which force is generated in the sarcomere is unknown. It seems likely that none of the theories proposed thus far is correct in all details. The cross-bridge theory appears to fail to satisfy stability criteria. This, to us, seems potentially a major difficulty, as any theory obviously needs to be compatible with established physical phenomena. Iwazumi's theory does not take into account some of the newer information concerning the dynamics of contractile protein structure (see Perry, this book). On the other hand, it is stable, simple, and seems compatible with much biochemical and biophysical data. For these reasons we are attracted to the principle of force generation outlined by Iwazumi, although not necessarily all the details of the theory.

Finally, it seems premature to test these theories on cardiac muscle. Until myocardial mechanics can be studied at the sarcomere level, we feel it will not be fruitful to try to relate cardiac mechanics to molecular theories.

REFERENCES

Blinks, J.R. (1970). Factors influencing the prolongation of active state by stretch in isolated heart muscle. Fed. Proc. 29, 2046.

Cleworth, D.R. and Edman, K.A.P. (1972). Changes in sarcomere length during isometric tension development in frog skeletal muscle. J. Physiol. 227, 1-17.

Davies, R.E. (1963). A molecular theory of muscle contraction: calcium dependent contractions with hydrogen bond formation plus ATP dependent extension of part of the myosin-acting cross-bridges. Nature, 199, 1068.

Ebashi, S. (1972). Calcium ions and muscle contraction. Nature, 240, 217.

Elliott, G.F., Lowy, J. and Millman, B.M. (1967). Low angle X-ray diffraction studies of living muscle during contraction. J. Mol. Biol. 25, 31.

Elliott, G.F., Lowy, J. and Worthington, C.R. (1963). An X-ray and light diffraction study of the filament lattice of striated muscle in the living state and in rigor. J. Mol. Biol. 6, 295.

Elliott, G.F. and Matsubara, I. (1972). The constant-volume behaviour of the myofilament lattice in frog skeletal muscle: studies of skinned fibers by X-ray and light duffraction. J. Physiol. 226, 88-89.

Elliott, G.F., Rome, E.M. and Spencer, M. (1970). A type of contraction hypothesis applicable to all muscles. Nature, 226, 417.

Ford, L.E., Huxley, A.F. and Simmons, R.M. (1974). Mechanism of early tension recovery after a quick release in tetanized muscle fibres. Proc. Physiol. Soc. March, 42-43P (J. Physiol. in Press).

Gale, H.H. and Davies, K.M. (1973). Transverse forces in skeletal muscle. Fed. Proc. March, 881 Abs.

Gordon, A.M., Huxley, A.F. and Julian, F.J. (1966). The variation in isometric tension with sarcomere length in vertebrate muscle fibers. J. Physiol. 184, 170-192.

Hill, A.V. (1938). The heat of shortening and the dynamic constants of muscle. Proc. Roy. Soc. B. 126, 136-195.

Hoyle, G., McNeill, P.A. and Selverston, A.I. (1973). Ultrastructure of barnacle giant muscle fibres. J. Cell. Biol. 56, 74-91.

Huxley, A.F. (1957). Muscle structure and theories of contraction. Progr. Biophys. 7, 257-318.

Huxley, A.F. and Niedergerke, R. (1954). Structural changes in muscle during contraction. Nature, 173, 971.

Huxley, A.F. and Simmons, R.M. (1970). J. Physiol. 208, 52-53 P.

Huxley, A.F. and Simmons, R.M. (1971). Proposed mechanism of force generation in striated muscle. Nature, 233, 533-538.

Huxley, H.E. (1969). The mechanism of muscular contraction. Science, 164, 1356-1366.

Huxley, H.E. and Hanson, J. (1954). Changes in the cross strations of muscle during contraction and stretch and their natural interpretation. Nature, 173, 973.

Ingels, N.P. and Thompson, N.P. (1966). An electrokinematic theory of muscle contraction. Nature, 211, 1032.

Iwazumi, (1970). A new field theory of muscle contraction, thesis, University of Pennsylvania.

Jewell, B.R., and Wilkie, D.R. (1958). An analysis of the mechanical components in frog's striated muscle. J. Physiol. 143, 515-540.

Johnson, E.A. et al. Light diffraction of cardiac muscle: sarcomere motion during contraction. CIBA symposium on "Physiological Basis of Starling's Law of the Heart". In Press.

Julian, F. (1971). The effect of calcium on the force-velocity relation of briefly glycernated frog muscle fibers. J. Physiol. 218, 117-145.

Leyton, R.A. and Sonnenblick, E.H. (1971). The sarcomere as the basis of Starling's law of the heart in the left and right ventricles. Meth. Achievm. Exp. Path. 5, 22-59.

Meiss, R.A. and Sonnenblick, E.H. (1972). Controlled shortening in heart muscle: velocity-force and active-state properties. Amer. J. Physiol. 3, 630-639.

Miller, A. and Tregear, R.T. (1970). Evidence concerning cross-bridge attachment during muscle contraction. Nature, 226, 1060-1061.

Nilsson, E. (1972). Influence of muscle length on the mechanical parameters of myocardial contraction. Acta Physiol. Scand. 85, 1.

Noble, M.I.M., Bowen, T.E. and Hefner, L.L. (1969). Force-velocity relationship of cat cardiac muscle studied by isotonic and quick-release techniques. Circ. Res. 24, 821-833.

Noble, M.I.M. and Else, W. (1972). Re-examination of the applicability of the Hill model of muscle to cat myocardium. Circ. Res. 31, 580-589.

Podolsky, R.J. and Nolan, A.C. (1973). Cold Spring Harb. Symp. Quant. Biol. 37, 661-668.

Pollack, G.H. and Huntsman, L.L. Sarcomere length - active force relations in living mammalian cardiac muscle. Amer. J. Physiol. In Press.

Pollack, G.H., Huntsman, L.L. and Verdugo, P. (1972). Cardiac muscle models: an over extension of series elasticity? Circ. Res. 31, 569-579.

Rüdel, R. and Taylor, S.R. (1971). Striated muscle fibers: facilitation of contraction of short lengths by caffeine. Science, 172, 387-388.

Taylor, S.R. and Rudel, R. (1970). Striated muscle fibers: inactivation of contraction induced by shortening. Science, 167, 882-884.

The Role of Cyclic AMP in the Adrenergic Control of the Heart

ALBERT WOLLENBERGER

Central Institute of Heart and Circulatory Regulation Research,
Academy of Sciences of the DDR,
German Democratic Republic.

INTRODUCTION

In 1965, when a limited number of tissues had become known that responded to certain hormones with an increase in their level of cyclic AMP - in the meantime the number of such tissues and hormones has multiplied - Sutherland et al., (1965) formulated his famous 2-messenger theory of hormone action, which in its present-day version is illustrated in Fig. 1. The hormone - it can also be a neurotransmitter substance or another extracellular signal - meets at the surface of its target cells its specific receptor, so far as we know a protein which in some way, probably through phospholipids, communicates with adenylate

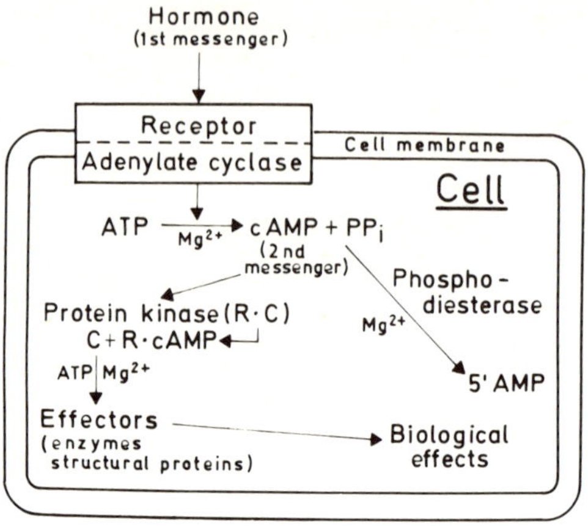

Figure 1. The two-messenger system of hormone action.

cyclase, the enzyme which in the presence of Mg^{2+} catalyzes the reaction: ATP ⟶ cyclic AMP + inorganic pyrophosphate. The interaction of hormone and its receptor triggers or increases the activity of the cyclase and therewith the formation of cyclic AMP, the intracellular (second) messenger. According to a widely accepted theory, promulgated by Greengard and Kuo, (1970), the cyclic AMP formed activates one or several cyclic AMP-dependent protein kinases. This type of enzyme consists of two subunits, a regulatory (R) and a catalytic (C) one (Brostrom et al., 1970). The R.C complex is catalytically inactive. What cyclic AMP does is to dissociate these two subunits by attaching itself as an allosteric effector to the regulatory subunit. C, the catalytic subunit, can then exert its function, namely, the transfer of the terminal phosphate of ATP to proteins. So far as we know, this phosphate transfer consists in the formation of phosphoester bonds with serine and also threonine residues of the polypeptide chains of these protein substrates. The ensueing changes in the properties of the various protein substrates (enzymes, structural proteins) manifest themselves physiologically as increases or decreases in enzyme activity, changes in permeability, and other characteristic hormone effects.

The stimulation of adenylate cyclase and protein kinases has the consequence that for every hormone molecule that becomes effective, many cyclic AMP molecules are formed and still many more terminal phosphate groups of ATP are transferred to the protein substrates of the kinases. This amplification factor can partly explain why minute amounts of hormones can bring about dramatic physiological changes.

Another group of enzymes as ubiquitous in nature as adenylate cyclase, namely cyclic AMP phosphodiesterases, subject to inhibition by compounds such as theophylline and papaverine, converts cyclic AMP, by opening its phosphate ring, into the physiologically inactive or differently active 5'-AMP. Still another enzyme group, the phosphoprotein phosphatases, terminate through protein dephosphorylation the hormone effects mediated by cyclic AMP. There still are hormones that have not yet been shown to exert their action via cyclic AMP as their intracellular mediator. Furthermore, there may be, and probably are, hormones that are using cyclic AMP as a second messenger for some but not for all of their actions. Finally, it is possible that protein phosphorylation does not constitute the sole mechanism of action of cyclic AMP in animal cells.

After these general introductory remarks which are intended to facilitate the understanding of some of the points to be considered later in this presentation, let me come to the subject of cyclic AMP and the heart, an organ which during each phase of its beat is under neural and hormonal control. In keeping with the theme of this session I shall restrict myself to a discussion of the role, or possible role, of cyclic AMP in the adrenergic control of the heart, exerted through the transmitter substance of the cardiac sympathetic nerves, noradrenaline in mammals, and through adrenomedullary hormones, mainly adrenaline. These catecholamines, together with the parasympathetic neurotransmitter, acetylcholine, are, after all, the most important extrinsic chemical regulators of cardiac cellular activity. By the term "extrinsic" is meant a regulation that modulates the more elementary "intrinsic" regulation of the electrical and mechanical activity of the myocardial fibers which is achieved by the movement of the inorganic cations - Na^+, K^+, and Ca^{2+} - across the cell membrane and by the displacement of bound Ca^{2+} ions at the cell surface and inside the cell and which is superimposed upon the control of enzyme activity through changes in the intracellular concentrations of substrates and allosteric effectors. This neurohumoral and hormonal control provides for a rapid and delicate adjustment of cardiac performance to the needs of the organism. Other hormones and hormone-like substances, such as thyroid hormone, corticosteroids, prostaglandins, histamine, and glucagon are likewise capable of influencing cardiac functional and metabolic activity (the latter two compounds probably only in pharmacological concentrations), exerting their effects either directly or by supporting the action of the catecholamines, noradrenaline and adrenaline. Space does not permit to discuss these effects and interrelationships. It is worth mentioning, however, that cyclic AMP has been implicated, or suspected to be involved as an intracellular mediator in the cardiac action of most of these hormones (Epstein et al., 1971).

CYCLIC AMP AND ADRENERGIC STIMULATION OF GLYCOGENOLYSIS

There is little doubt that the most prominent metabolic effect of the catecholamines on the heart, the acceleration of glycogen breakdown, is mediated in the cytoplasm of the cardiac cells, in the presence of Ca^{2+} ions, by the second hormonal messenger, cyclic AMP, the formation of which is induced or accelerated when membrane-bound adenylate cyclase is stimulated by these hormones, or to be more explicit, by their interaction with the β-adrenoreceptor. Theoretically, an increase in the level of cyclic AMP in heart muscle exposed to a catecholamine could also be brought about by inhibition of cyclic AMP phosphodiesterase, the enzyme catalyzing the hydrolysis of cyclic AMP to 5'-AMP, and by slowing of the passage of cyclic AMP from the cell into the extracellular space and into the circulation. However, there is no evidence that catecholamines affect phosphodiesterase, except at unphysiologically high concentration (Goren and Rosen, 1972), and it is very unlikely that a change in the rate of efflux of cyclic AMP could materially affect the tissue cyclic AMP level in the short time interval interceding between exposure to the hormone and completion of the rise in cyclic AMP.

The currently held view about the pathway of the catecholamine effect on myocardial glycogenolysis is depicted in Fig.2 in form of a

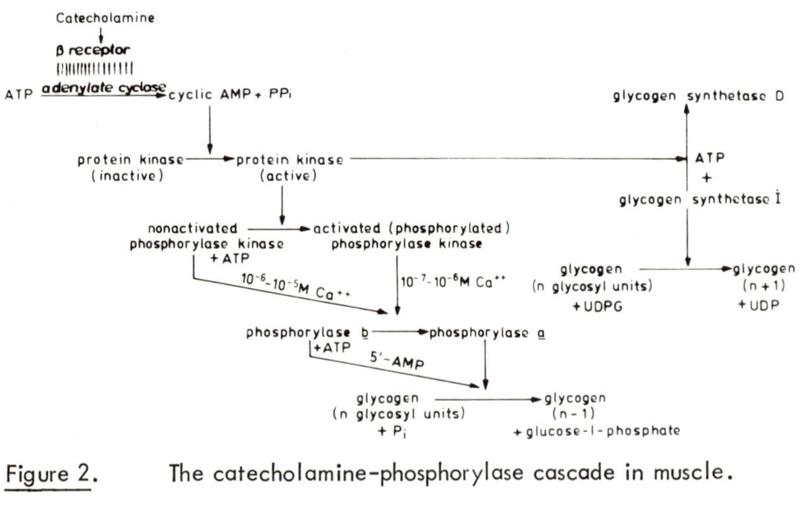

Figure 2. The catecholamine-phosphorylase cascade in muscle.

reaction cascade, which nature has invented as a device for the amplification of a weak initial signal. The sequence of these reactions has been rather firmly established in skeletal muscle, mainly through the work of Edwin Krebs and his collaborators (Brostrom et al., 1970 ; Krebs et al., 1968) ; it remains to be fully documented in heart muscle, but there is little reason to think that the cascade does not operate there. The initial signal in Fig.2, a catecholamine, stimulates, after its interaction with the β-receptor, adenylate cyclase, causing thereby an acceleration of the formation of cyclic AMP. Cyclic AMP stimulates, by the mechanism outlined in the Fig.1, a protein kinase which catalyzes the phosphorylation of non-activated phosphorylase kinase and of active glycogen synthetase (the glucose-6-phosphate-independent or I form), converting the former enzyme into the active form and the latter enzyme into the inactive (glucose-6-phosphate-dependent or D form) (Soderling et al., 1970). The activated phsophorylase kinase in turn catalyzes, in the presence of 2 - 5 x 10^{-7}M Ca^{2+}, the phosphorylation and activation of glycogen phosphorylase, i.e. the transformation of phosphorylase <u>b</u> to <u>a</u>. This results in the acceleration of the breakdown of glycogen to glucose-1-phosphate, at the same time as glycogen synthesis is slowed by the conversion of the synthetase from the L to the D form. Let me point out that also the nonphosphorylated, nonactivated phosphorylase kinase can be active, provided that the cytoplasmic free Ca^{2+} concentration reaches a level of 10^{-6} to 10^{-5}M (Brostrom et al., 1971), which is the case in muscle, including heart muscle, during the activation phase of contraction. In any event, this enzyme is absolutely calcium-dependent. What phosphorylation does, is to increase its calcium sensitivity. The phosphorylation of phosphorylase kinase, discovered in 1968 by Walsh, Perkins, and Krebs, was the first known case of a cyclic AMP-dependent phosphorylation of a protein. This by now classical discovery provided the impetus to studies from which evolved the theory (Greengard and Kuo, 1970), mentioned before, that protein phosphorylation constitutes a general mechanism of action of cyclic AMP.

A similar reaction cascade, started by catecholamines in adipose tissue, leads to the mobilization of free fatty acids. Here it is the hormone-sensitive lipase which is phosphorylated and activated by a cyclic AMP-dependent protein kinase, incidentally directly, without the intervention of a lipase kinase that would correspond to phosphorylase kinase in the hormone-phosphorylase cascade (Hutunnen and Steinberg, 1971). A catecholamine-lipase cascade has not yet been proven to exist in heart muscle, but its existence can be surmised by analogy and from the fact that heart muscle responds to catecholamines and also to dibutyryl cyclic AMP with increased triglyceride mobilization and release of free fatty acids (Christian et al., 1969 ; Crass, 1973) , which in this tissue constitute an important source of metabolic energy (Opie, 1968).

PHOSPHORYLASE ACTIVATION AND POSITIVE INOTROPIC EFFECT

Aerobic Myocardium. At one time it was thought possible (Haugaard and Hess, 1965 ; Hess and Haugaard, 1958) that the β-adrenoreceptor and cyclic AMP-mediated activation of the myocardial phosphorylase system and the resulting acceleration of glycogenolysis and glycolytic energy production may directly and causally be related to the increase in myocardial contractile force brought about by catecholamines. However this idea became untenable when it was shown that small doses of catecholamines could have positive inotropic effects on the myocardium without increasing phosphorylase *a* levels (Mayer, et al., 1963) and that with higher doses the peak of the positive inotropic response preceded, under certain conditions, the maximum of the activation of phosphorylase (Cheung and Williamson, 1965 ; Drummond et al., 1966 ; Drummond et al., 1964 ; Øye, 1965 ; Robison et al., 1965 ; Williamson and Jamieson, 1965) ; on the other hand, the rise in cyclic AMP occurred even slightly earlier than the increase in contractility (Cheung and Williamson, 1965 ; Drummond et al., 1966 ; Drummond and Hemmings, 1973 ; Kukovetz et al., 1973 ; Namm and Mayer, 1968 ; Robison et al., 1965). It thus seems clear that activation of phosphorylase is not a prerequisite for the positive inotropic action of the catecholamines, at least not in aerobically contracting myocardium. Neither is the increase in contractile force a necessary condition for the phosphorylase-activating effect. But energy production stimulated by catecholamines may be needed for the support of the increased contractile activity. As Haugaard et al.,(1973) have stated, an adequate supply of ATP is a condition required for the full expression of the positive inotropic effect of the catecholamines on the heart, particularly if this effect should be longer lasting.

Ischaemic myocardium. In emergency situations, such as sudden coronary insufficiency, paroxysmal tachycardia, or severe physical exertion, in which the availability of oxygen to the myocardium does not meet, or not quite meet, the oxygen demands, catecholamine-induced and cyclic AMP-mediated activation of phsophorylase and acceleration of glycolysis may be instrumental and even essential in helping the muscle to replenish its supply of ATP needed for contraction. An example of this is given by the data in Fig.3, which represents the biochemical response of dog myocardium to sudden arrest of the coronary flow. In this situation, as was shown in our laboratory (Shahab et al., 1969), there is a rapid mobilization of endogenous cardiac noradrenaline, which appears to be a direct effect of acute myocardial ischemia independent of cardiac sympathetic nerve activity, and it has the following consequencies (Wollenberger et al., 1969) : First a rise in cardiac cyclic AMP, followed by a rise in activated phosphorylase kinase and then phosphorylase _a_, and by a rise in

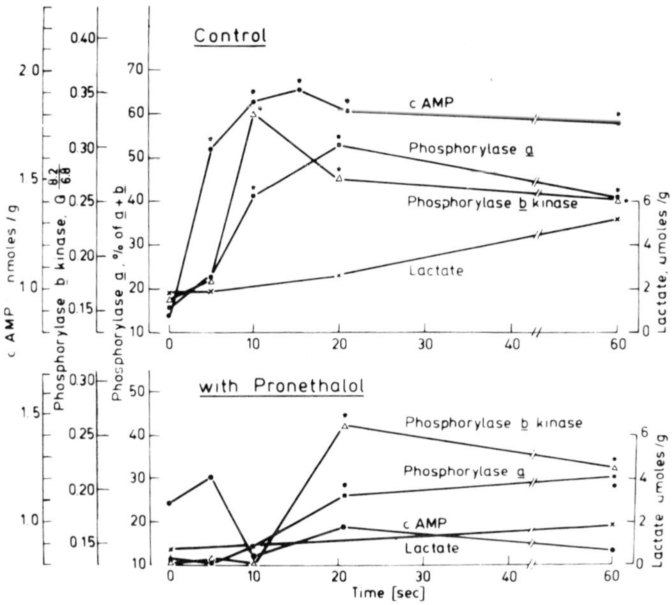

Figure 3. Some biochemical responses of dog myocardium to arrest of blood flow (Wollenberger and Krause, 1973). Open-chest dogs, pentobarbitone anesthesia, artificial respiration. At 0 sec, the ascending aorta was cut. Small subepicardial pieces of the left ventricle were consecutively and almost instantly frozen *in situ* at 0 sec and at different times thereafter. The asterisks denote values which differ from the respective 0-sec values at a level of significance of 5% or lower. Replacement of the cyclic AMP assay procedure used in these experiments by a protein binding assay yielded values which lie approximately 30% below those shown here.

lactate production. The predominantly adrenergic initiation of these changes is also documented by the finding (Fig.4) that the rise in cyclic AMP was abolished and the increases in activated phosphorylase kinase, phosphorylase _a_, and lactate were delayed and slowed when animals were pretreated with β-blockers. Fig.4 shows this inhibition for cardiac cyclic AMP and phosphorylase _a_ in dogs given pronethalol. We also found the same type of inhibited biochemical response to sudden myocardial ischemia in animals with cardiac hypertrophy due to aortic constriction or renal hypertension in which the cardiac noradrenaline stores were severely depleted (Wollenberger et al., 1973).

CYCLIC AMP AND THE ACTION OF CATECHOLAMINES ON CARDIAC FUNCTION

After this excursion into cardiac pathophysiology let me turn, or return, to the main topic of my talk, which concerns a question that for some time has been moving the minds of quite a few cardiac physiologists and pharmacologists, namely whether or not cyclic AMP acts as a mediator of the effects of the catecholamines on the functional properties of the heart, in the first place contractility and automaticity.

Chronotropic Action

Because of the small dimensions of the pacemaker regions of the heart and because of difficulties in precisely localizing them macroscopically for the purpose of isolation there have been few attempts to

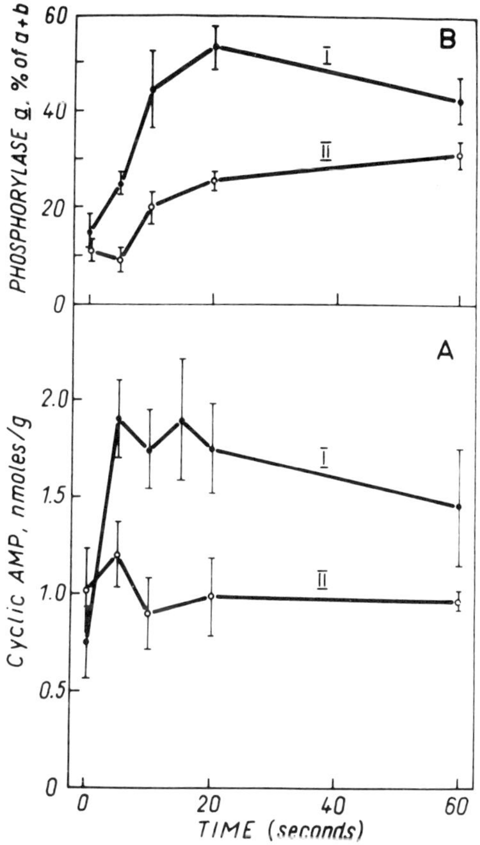

Figure 4. Cyclic AMP and phosphorylase a levels in the left ventricle of the dog before and after arrest of the coronary blood flow (Wollenberger et al., 1969). I : Dogs not treated with pronethalol ; II : dogs treated with pronethalol, 7 mg/kg given intravenously 20 min prior to "0 sec". Experimental conditions were the same as those described in the legend of Fig. 3. The points and vertical bars represent the means ± standard errors.

apply biochemical techniques to the study of the possible role of cyclic AMP in the positive chronotropic action of the catecholamines. Little information exists as yet on the levels of cyclic AMP and on adenylate cyclase activity in cardiac pacemaker tissue and cells, and none on cyclic nucleotide phosphodiesterase. Potentiation of the heart beat accelerating effect of catecholamines by phosphodiesterase inhibitors could be an indicator for an involvement of cyclic AMP in this effect. Adenylate cyclase activity in particles prepared from cultures of new-born rat heart cells in which many, if not the majority of myocardial cells may have regained the facility of autorhythmicity that was suppressed at an early stage of embryogenesis (Wollenberger, 1964) was stimulated by adrenaline to about the same extent as in particulate preparations of the new-born rat heart, namely, by maximally about 75%, as compared to a 150% stimulation in particles of the adult rat heart (P. Karczewski, unpublished). The basal activity of the enzyme in the cultured heart cell particles was only one third of the activity in the particles of the fresh new-born heart. The latter particles did not differ significantly from those of the adult heart with respect to basal adenylate cyclase activity. A 15-minute exposure to 2×10^{-7} M adrenaline caused a 230% elevation in the cyclic AMP level of the cultured heart cells in the absence of theophylline and a 470% elevation in its presence (R. Irmler, unpublished). This is a concentration which also caused a marked increase in the rate of beat of the cells. This increase could be prevented by β-adrenoreceptor blockers (propranolol and MJ 1999), but not by the α -blocker phentolamine. In homogenized Purkinje fibres of the adult dog heart propranolol blocked the stimulatory action of positive chronotropic concentrations of adrenaline on adenylate cyclase activity (Dhalla et al., 1973). It was suggested that the adenylate cyclase system may be involved in the regulation of automaticity by β-adrenergic amines. More specifically, it was proposed (McNaughton and Noble, 1973), on the basis of voltage clamp experiments with sheep Purkinje fibres, that a reduction in the intracellular concentration of Ca^{2+} ions induced by adrenaline and involving cyclic AMP would reduce the positive charge density on the inside of the plasma membrane, causing a depolarizing shift responsible for the acceleration of the cardiac pacemaker.

N^6-monobutyryl cyclic AMP, added to superfused, electrically driven calf Purkinje fibres in a concentration of 2 mM, resembled noradrenaline in its effect on the configuration of the action potential (Tsien et al., 1972). The same was found to be the case following addition of N^6, 2'-0-dibutyryl cyclic AMP to spontaneously contracting dog heart Purkinje fibres (Danilo et al., 1972). This compound was also found to resemble adrenaline in its ability to restore spontaneous electrical activity in arrested cardiac pacemaker tissue (Tuganowski et al., 1973). These butyryl derivatives of cyclic AMP are more lipophilic, and can better enter the cell, than the natural parent compound, in addition of being more resistant to cyclic AMP phosphodiesterases (Drummond and Hemmings, 1972 ; Henion et al., 1967 ; Kaukel and Hilz, 1972). The monobutyryl derivative possesses intrinsic biological activity as activator of cyclic AMP-dependent protein kinases (Rebhuhn and Villar-Palasi, 1973). Thus partial deacylation of the dibutyryl derivative inside the cell to yield the N^6-monobutyryl compound may suffice to evoke biological activity. In spontaneously active calf Purkinje fibres intracellular iontophoretic injection of cyclic AMP caused changes similar to those produced by adrenaline, i.e. a positive chronotropic effect characterized by a steeper pacemaker depolarization and a briefer plateau phase of the action potential (Tsien, 1973). Iontophoretic injection of 5'-AMP was without effect. These findings were taken as constituting evidence for a mediator function of cyclic AMP in the electrical effects of adrenaline on the heart.

That cyclic AMP may be involved in the positive chronotropic cardiac action of the catecholamines had been suggested earlier (Krause et al., 1970 ; Kukovetz and Poch, 1970) and was subsequently confirmed (Boder and Johnson, 1972 ; Dhalla et al., 1973 ; Drummond and Hemmings, 1972) by reports that dibutyryl cyclic AMP was capable of increasing the frequency of beat in isolated cultured heart cells and in the intact heart. Confidence in these findings, however, was somewhat weakened by the inability of other authors (Chiba et al., 1972 ; Gartner and Vahovny, 1972 ; Wildenthal, 1973) to observe a positive chronotropic effect of dibutyryl cyclic AMP on the heart.

Inotropic Action

The chief functional characteristic of the bulk of the cardiac muscle mass, which lends itself more easily to biochemical analysis than the cardiac pacemaker regions, is its ability to contract. Many investigations over the last ten years have been concerned with the question, whether or not the contraction-strengthening effect of the catecholamines on the myocardium is mediated by cyclic AMP. The results of these studies have been far from unequivocal and opinion on the question at issue is sharply divided.

Evidence Against a Direct Participation of Cyclic AMP in the Positive Inotropic Cardiac Action of the Catecholamines

A number of investigators believe that stimulation of adenylate cyclase by catecholamines is an effect which is not directly related to the positive inotropic cardiac action of these hormones. This concept was first clearly put forth by Ebashi,(1969) and is illustrated in the diagram shown in Fig.5, which is a drawing taken from Ebashi's paper. A basic phenomenon of cardiac pharmacology expressed in this figure is that the action of the catecholamines on myocardial contractility, like that of a number of other positive inotropic agents, is tied to their ability to increase

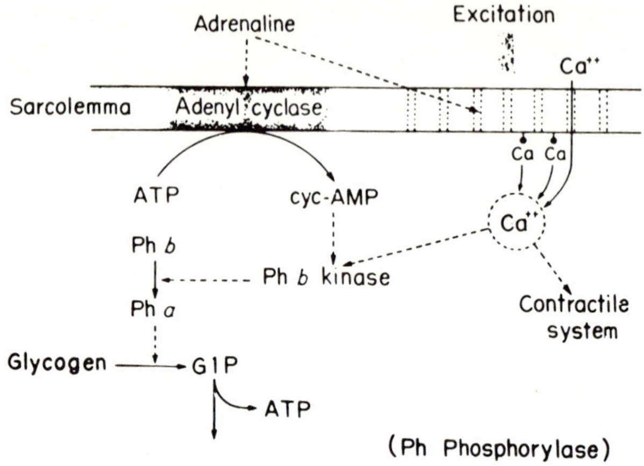

Figure 5. Model of a parallel involvement of cyclic AMP and Ca^{2+} in the effects of adrenaline on the heart muscle cell. From Ebashi, (1969).

in the myoplasm during each contraction cycle the amount of ionized calcium that functions as activator of the contractile system. It was shown over 10 years ago by Grossman and Furchgott, (1964) and by Reuter, (1965) that the positive inotropic action of adrenaline on the heart is associated with an increase in the influx of extracellular Ca^{2+} into the myocardial fibres during depolarization. This is schematically shown in Fig. 5 by the broken line channels in the membrane; the figure also pictures superficially bound Ca^{2+} that is released into the cell interior on excitation, an idea elaborated upon by Langer, (Langer 1971, 1973) who proposes that this is the way in which extracellular

Ca^{2+} passes into the myocardial cell. At any rate, Ca^{2+} entering the myoplasm during excitation across and from the cell surface is, in the view expressed in Fig.5, the second messenger of adrenaline for its positive inotropic action on the myocardium. This Ca^{2+} is at the same time pictured in the figure as co-operating with the cyclic AMP formed under the influence of adrenaline in the stimulation of phosphorylase kinase activity, an enzyme that, as will be recalled from Fig.2, has an absolute requirement for Ca^{2+}. The kinetics of phosphorylase kinase are such that even a lowering of the Ca^{2+} requirement through phosphorylation (apparent K_m for Ca^{2+} of 2×10^{-7}M at pH 8.2) will only allow for about 20 per cent of the full catalytic activity of the enzyme when it is brought into contact with Ca^{2+}-sequestring sarcoplasmic reticulum in a reconstituted muscular system (Brostrom et al., 1971). Thus the adrenaline-induced and cyclic AMP-mediated phosphorylation of phosphorylase kinase at the free intracellular Ca^{2+} concentration prevailing in (heart) muscle during relaxation does not become effective in terms of enhanced catalytic activity unless there is a rise in cellular Ca^{2+} concentration above the resting level. On the other hand, a rise in the cellular cyclic AMP level is not required, according to the model shown in Fig.5, for the Ca^{2+}-mediated positive inotropic effect of adrenaline. A similar model of the mechanism of the positive inotropic cardiac action of the catecholamines and of its link, through Ca^{2+}, to the glycogenolytic action of the hormone has been presented by Rasmussen, (1970).

These models of parallel catecholamine actions on myocardial contractility on the one hand and cyclic AMP levels and glycogenolysis on the other hand have received substantial backing from several studies in which instances of a dissociation of the positive inotropic and the cyclic AMP-elevating effects of catecholamines were observed.

The first such case reported was the failure of the weak β-blocker, N-isopropylmethoxamine, to inhibit the positive inotropic response in noradrenaline-treated heart muscle in a dose (10 μg/ml) which suppressed the stimulation of cyclic AMP formation and also the activation of phosphorylase (Shanfeld et al., 1969). However, since this dose produces a depression of myocardial contractile force, the possible influence of this depression on the biochemical responses should be taken into account before concluding that the effects of catecholamines on myocardial contractility and cyclic AMP levels can be dissociated by N-isopropylmethoxamine (Mayer, 1970 ; Wastila et al., 1972). Furthermore, that component of the positive inotropic action of noradrenaline on the heart which may be triggered by stimulation of α -adrenoreceptors (Govier, 1968) would not be expected to be inhibited by a B-blocker (Robison et al., 1971). In a later study (Brooker, 1971) the positive inotropic cardiac effects of adrenaline and noradrenaline could not be dissociated by isopropylmethoxamine from increased myocardial cyclic AMP levels.

Alpha agonism may also have been the reason why in experiments reported by Benfey, (1971) the positive inotropic cardiac response to phenylephrine was not parallel by a rise in cyclic AMP. Since α -adrenergic activity may cause a fall in cyclic AMP (Robison et al., 1971), it is conceivable (McNeill et al., 1972) that the α - and β-effects of phenylephrine on adenylate cyclase may have cancelled each other, with the result that the cardiac cyclic AMP level did not change. In the studies of McNeill and Verma, (1973) and Drummond and Hemmings, (1973), however, phenylephrine produced in perfused heart preparations dose-dependent increases in both contractile force and cyclic AMP as well as phosphorylase _a_ levels. In other experiments (Øye and Osnes, 1973) in which the positive inotropic response of perfused hearts to phenylephrine was accompanied by a modest rise in cardiac cyclic AMP, the β-antagonist propranolol abolished the rise in cyclic AMP, but not the positive inotropic response.

In Benfey's (Benfey, 1971) study dopamine likewise failed to stimulate cyclic AMP synthesis in ventricular slices in concentrations having strong inotropic effects on isolated atria. Experiments on isolated perfused heart indicate that the cyclic AMP content of the tissue can be raised by dopamine, though not to the same extent as by administration of isoproterenol or noradrenaline (Øye and Osnes, 1973). These results may be viewed in the light of the finding (Bilezikian and Aurbach, 1973 ; Schramm et al., 1972) that the absence of the β-hydroxyl group in the side chain that distinguishes the structure of dopamine from that of noradrenaline leads to a considerable weakening of the stimulating effect on adenylate cyclase without greatly affecting binding to the putative β-receptor.

Not readily refutable arguments against a participation of cyclic AMP in the contractile response of the heart to catecholamines have been furnished by the studies of Langslet and Øye,(1970 ; Øye and Langslet,(1972) and of Kjekshus et al.,(1971). In some of these studies cellular permeability was increased in isolated perfused hearts by lowering the temperature (Langslet and Øye, 1970) and by addition of dimethyl sulphoxide to the perfusion fluid (Kjekshus et al., 1971). In both cases added cyclic AMP activated phsophorylase without increasing contractility, while the contractile response to adrenaline was preserved. In other experiments (Øye and Langslet, 1972) on perfused heart preparations beating under standard conditions, low concentrations of dibutyryl cyclic AMP activated phosphorylase, but had no effect on the contractile force. With higher concentrations the activation of phosphorylase preceded the onset of a positive inotropic effect by several minutes. Chlorpromazine, termed a "membrane stabilizer" (Øye and Langslet, 1972), suppressed the rise in cyclic AMP and greatly depressed the activation of phosphorylase brought about by low concentrations of isoprenaline without affecting the contractile force. Øye and Langslet,(1972) postulate that a "labilization" of the cell membrane by adrenaline would on the one hand result in the ionic changes which form the basis for the increase in contractility and other functional parameters and, on the other hand, would provide the stimulus for adenylate cyclase. This is an attractive proposition, because a change in the configuration of part of the plasma membrane may well constitute the mechanism whereby the signal generated by hormone-receptor interaction is transduced to stimulate amplifying elements in the membrane (e.g. adenylate cyclase, ion translocation systems) that yield the intracellular signal or signals (Birnbaumer et al., 1970 ; Hechter, 1971). Kjekshus et al., (1971) recall the hypothesis of Rasmussen and Tennenhouse,(1968), according to which hormonal stimulation of adenylate cyclase results in the formation of cyclic AMP and free Ca^{2+} from a postulated calcium-membrane-ATP complex. These Ca^{2+} ions rather than cyclic AMP would then be the primary signal for the augmentation of contractile strength. We may add that, if membrane-bound Ca^{2+} is in equilibrium with extracellular Ca^{2+}, this mechanism could account for the increased influx of the ion into the myocardial fibre under the influence of a catecholamine (see above). Cyclic AMP could then be assigned an auxiliary role in catecholamine inotropism

(Øye and Langslet, 1972) that would consist, among other actions, in accelerating glycolytic energy production helpful for the support of increased mechanical activity (Øye and Langslet, 1972).

Evidence in Support on an Obligatory Involvement of Cyclic AMP in the Positive Inotropic Cardiac Action of the Catecholamines

The other (and older) school of thought on the role of cyclic AMP in the action of catecholamines on cardiac contraction places the nucleotide right on the main road connecting the catecholamines and the augmented contractile response, as summarized by Nayler,(1967) in the following sequence: catecholamine ⟶ increased cyclic AMP ⟶ changed membrane permeability ⟶ increased uptake of Ca^{2+} ⟶ increased intracellular Ca^{2+} ⟶ augmented contraction. According to this concept the increase in Ca^{2+} influx and the resulting positive inotropic response are consequencies of a catecholamine-induced increase in cyclic AMP. A more alaborate scheme of the same basic concept has been presented by Kukovetz and Pöch, 1972) and is reproduced in Fig.6. It features the idea, which is becoming supported by experimental evidence, that the myocardial cell membrane is the seat of both hormone-sensitive adenylate cyclase (Drummond and Duncan, 1970 ; Tada et al., 1972 ; Williamson and Scarpa, 1973 ; Wollenberger et al., 1973), cyclic nucleotide phosphodiesterase (Campbell and Oliver, 1972 ; Kukovetz and Pöch, 1970), cyclic AMP-dependent protein kinase (Krause et al.,

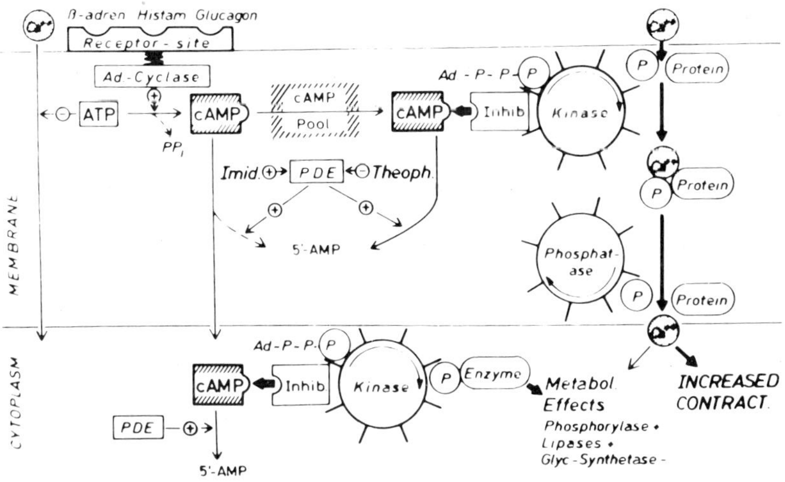

Figure 6. Model of a sequential involvement of cyclic AMP and Ca^{2+} in the action of β-adrenergic agonists (and other substances) on the contractile function of the myocardium. From Kukovetz and Pöch, (1972).

1973), phosphoprotein phosphatase (Krause et al., 1973), and also of the protein substrates of the two last-named enzymes. This membrane would thus possess all the equipment necessary for the formation and destruction of cyclic AMP as well as for its biological activity and the termination of that activity. The Ca^{2+} inward transport across the cell membrane is pictured, as in Fig. 5, as an essential site for hormonal regulation of myocardial contractility, but in contrast to the model in

Fig.5, cyclic AMP formed in response to hormone-receptor interaction acts, via a membrane-bound cyclic AMP-dependent protein kinase, on Ca^{2+} inward flow. This action is visualized in a still speculative manner as the operation of a phosphorylation - dephosphorylation cycle geared to the cardiac cycle in a manner quite analogous to that of the ATP-driven sodium pump. However, it is possible that the phosphorylated state of the protein substrate (s) is continuously maintained as long as the functional effects of the catecholamines are manifested, which could be the case for several minutes. It seems preferable at present to be rather non-committal about the way in which cyclic AMP-induced stimulation of membrane-bound protein kinase might affect the inward flow of Ca^{2+} (Will, et al., 1973). In its view of the co-operative action of cyclic AMP and Ca^{2+} on the phosphorylase system in the cytosol the model in Fig.6 is in agreement with that in Fig.2.

A relationship between cyclic AMP and Ca^{2+} not immediately evident from Fig.6 derives from the fact that cardiac cyclic AMP phosphodiesterase is activated (Teo and Wang, 1973) and cardiac adenylate cyclase is inhibited (Drummond and Duncan, 1970) by Ca^{2+}. At least in the case of the phosphodiesterase the effective concentrations of Ca^{2+} are low enough to be of potential physiological significance (Teo and Wang, 1973). There may thus exist a feedback mechanism whereby a cyclic AMP-induced temporary increase in the amount of

Ca^{2+} with which these two enzymes could come into contact, would cause an acceleration of cyclic AMP destruction and perhaps also a slowing of the formation of more cyclic AMP. This mechanism may play a role in the periodic oscillation of the cyclic AMP level that has been found in frog myocardium to be associated with the contraction cycle (Brooker, 1973 ; Wollenberger et al., 1973).

The model in Fig.4 draws much of its support from the fact that Sutherland's (Sutherland et al., 1968) 4 criteria for judging whether a given hormone effect is mediated by cyclic AMP have been met for catecholamines and cardiac contraction. As discussed by Sutherland et al.,(1968), adenylate cyclase in broken cell preparations was stimulated by low, inotropically effective concentrations, the inotropic response was associated with an increase in cyclic AMP, and it was potentiated by inhibition of cyclic AMP breakdown. In the intervening time the fourth criterion, reproduction of hormonal action by added cyclic AMP or one of its derivatives, has partly and possibly fully been satisfied. The N^6, 2'-0-dibutyryl derivative of cyclic AMP was found (Ahren et al., 1971 ; Bertelli et al., 1972 ; Boder and Johnson, 1972 ; Crass, 1973 ; Cutiletta et al., 1973 ; Dhalla et al., 1973 ; Drummond and Hemmings, 1972 ; Haas and Gokel, 1970 ; Kobayashi et al., 1971 ; Kukovetz and Pöch, 1970 ; Meinertz et al., 1972 ; Meinertz et al., 1973 ; Skelton et al., 1970) to provoke a positive inotropic response and, furthermore, to mimic the inotropic action of adrenaline both with respect to changes in certain parameters of contractility (maximal tension, rate of tension development) (Morad and Rellet, 1972 ; Skelton et al., 1970) and with respect to its magnitude and time course as influenced by the extracellular Ca^{2+} concentration (Meinertz et al., 1973). However, as pointed out in the preceding section, whereas adrenaline increases contractile force preferentially to activation of phosphorylase, dibutyryl cyclic AMP does not (Ahren et al., 1971) or even shows the reverse preference (Øye and Langslet, 1972). Furthermore, the ability of adrenaline to speed relaxation and to overcome KCl contracture was not reflected in the action of dibutyryl cyclic AMP on the frog heart (Morad and Rellet, 1972). In cultured monolayers of spontaneously beating rat heart cells the relaxation-accelerating action of adrenaline was clearly mimicked by dibutyryl cyclic AMP (Warbanow and Wollenberger, 1974). Another very significant parallelism between adrenaline and butyryl derivatives of cyclic AMP was established by the findings that the latter, like adrenaline, increase in mammalian cardiac muscle Ca^{2+} inward current (Tsien et al., 1972) and the rate of $^{45}Ca^{2+}$ uptake (Meinertz et al., 1973).

It also looks as if the fourth criterion of Sutherland (Sutherland et al., 1968) may have been met in a cell-free system of heart muscle. In a microsomal fraction of dog heart homogenate, stated to represent principally sarcoplasmic reticulum, in which adrenaline and also glucagon stimulated adenylate cyclase activity and increased Ca^{2+} binding (oxalate absent) and Ca^{2+} uptake (oxalate present), the latter effects were also obtained on addition of cyclic AMP. I am referring to the work of Entman et al.,(1969), published 5 years ago and subsequently confirmed in part by some (Gillibrand and Wyse, 1971 ; Shinebourne et al., 1969 ; Shinebourne and White, 1970), though not by all (Sabatini-Smith, 1971 ; Sulakhe and Dhalla, 1970) authors dealing with this problem. Another interesting aspect of this work was that it apparently revealed the presence of adrenaline-sensitive, i.e. β-adrenoreceptor-associated adenylate cyclase in membranes of the cardiac sarcoplasmic reticulum. This finding was corroborated by further studies, based on controlled tissue fractionation, of the subcellular distribution of the enzyme in cardiac muscle (Katz et al., 1974 ; Sulakhe and Dhalla, 1973). Sulakhe and Dhalla estimated that about 12 per cent of the total cardiac adenylate cyclase is located in the sarcoplasmic reticulum. Cytochemical studies in our laboratory (Wollenberger et al., 1973) tend to support these findings, although our evidence for the presence of adrenaline-stimulated adenylate cyclase activity in elements of the sarcoplasmic reticulum is more clear-cut in white skeletal muscle than it is in heart muscle (Schulze and Wollenberger, in press).

CALCIUM BINDING AND UPTAKE BY ISOLATED CARDIAC MEMBRANES AND OTHER COMPONENTS AS INFLUENCED BY CYCLIC AMP-DEPENDENT PROTEIN PHOSPHYORYLATION

Sarcoplasmic Reticulum

Now if Ca^{2+} binding and uptake and perhaps other properties of cardiac membranes which display adenylate cyclase activity are altered by adrenaline and also directly by cyclic AMP, one would predict, on the basis of the protein kinase theory of cyclic AMP action (Greengard and Kuo, 1970), that such effects may be the consequence of a phosphorylation of membrane protein by cyclic AMP-dependent protein kinase(s). Kirchberger et al.,(1972) incubated dog heart microsomes rich in sarcoplasmic reticulum fragments in a medium containing, among other constituents, ATP, Mg^{2+}, and a partially purified cyclic AMP-dependent protein kinase from bovine heart, and observed on addition of cyclic AMP a stimulation of phsophate incorporation into a microsomal protein of molecular weight of 22,000 daltons and an acceleration of oxalate-dependent Ca^{2+} uptake into the microsomal vesicles. Ca^{2+} binding, measured in the absence of oxalate, was not affected by this treatment. Similar observations were made by other authors (La Raia et al., 1973 ; Rodnight and Weller, 1972 ; Wray et al., 1973) in sarcoplasmic reticulum-enriched subcellular heart muscle fractions exhibiting <u>endogenous</u> cyclic AMP-dependent protein kinase activity. It was concluded by Katz and Repke,(1973) that hormones such as the catecholamines, which stimulate the formation of cyclic AMP in the myocardium, ought to promote the translocation of Ca^{2+} ions from the myoplasm and their binding sites on troponin to the Ca^{2+} storage organelles, presumably the terminal cisternae of the sarcoplasmic reticulum. Such an effect could explain the acceleration of relaxation which is an important component of the action of the catecholamines on the cardiac contraction cycle (Morad and Rellet, 1972 ; Reiter, 1972). The positive inotropic action of these amines is then explained on the ground that after augmented Ca^{2+} storage more Ca^{2+} can be set free by excitation during the succeeding heart beats (Entman et al., 1969 ; Himms-Hagen, 1972 ; Katz and Repke, 1973). Both conclusions are somewhat speculative. In the first place it is not certain that the so-called uptake of Ca^{2+} ions by membrane vesicles in the presence of oxalate has a physiological correlate; according to Ebashi and Endo,(1968) this is not the case. Secondly, it is not certain that substances which enhance the ability of membrane structures to take up and bind Ca^{2+} ions necessarily contribute to an augmented release of these ions. It has been shown in microsomes from smooth muscle loaded with $^{45}Ca^{2+}$ that such substances inhibit the spontaneous release of this cation (Baudouin-Legros and Meyer, 1973). However, this release may not be representative of the Ca^{2+} release occurring after physiological excitation of intact myocardium.

Myofibrils

Troponin, the Ca^{2+}-binding regulatory protein of the myofibrils about which we have heard from Professor Perry (Perry, in press), has been phosphorylated in the test tube by a purified cyclic AMP-dependent protein kinase (Bailey and Villar-Palasi, 1971 ; Pratje and Heilmeyer, 1972) and also by a protein kinase tightly associated with the tropomyosin-troponin complex (Reddy et al., 1973). In one laboratory (Bailey and Villar-Palasi, 1971) it was the inhibitory and in another (Pratje and Heilmeyer, 1972) the tropomyosin-associated subunit (TNI and TNT, respectively) that served as phosphate acceptor. Both subunits could also be phosphorylated by phosphorylase kinase (Perry and Cole, 1973 ; Stull et al., 1972), the inhibitory subunit equally well by the non-phosphorylated, non-activated and by the phosphorylated, activated form of the enzyme (Stull et al., 1972), i.e. independently of cyclic AMP (see above). In none of these cases mentioned has it been shown that the Ca^{2+}-binding and regulatory properties of troponin were altered by phosphorylation. On the other hand, it was reported by Heilmeyer and Pratje,(1973) that phsophorylation of actin by a cyclic AMP-dependent protein kinase causes a four-fold increase in the Ca^{2+} sensitivity of actomyosin ATPase reconstituted from actin, myosin, and troponin. This effect, provided that it occurs in intact muscle, could be of physiological significance.

Cell Surface Membrane

In our laboratory, work is in progress which is closely related to some of the studies just discussed, but in which an attempt is made to focus attention more on the myocardial cell surface membrane. As we were told in the preceding session, the movement of Ca^{2+} across this membrane is of overwhelming importance to the regulation of myocardial contractile function, and as we shall undoubtedly hear in next presentation, the positive inotropic action of the sympathomimetic amines on heart muscle can be related to an increased Ca^{2+} influx during membrane depolarization (Grossman and Furchgott, 1964; Reuter, 1965). A corresponding increase in Ca^{2+} efflux, which serves to keep the cellular Ca^{2+} ion concentration constant, can be expected to be of relevance to the relaxing effect of these amines (Reuter, 1965). It is therefore of interest to know, whether and how the cyclic AMP - protein kinase system, as a possible intermediary in the effects of β-adrenergic sympathomimetic amines on myocardial contractile activity, may effect the interaction of the myocardial cell surface membrane with Ca^{2+}.

(a) Cyclic AMP-Stimulated Protein Phosphorylation

We have used different types of cardiac cell membrane or cell membrane-enriched preparations in this work, with more or less comparable results. In a first series of experiments (Wollenberger and Krause,

1973) a cell surface membrane preparation from pig myocardium, isolated by the method of Kono and Colowick, (1961) as applied to heart muscle by Portius and Repke, (1967) and kindly supplied by Dr. Portius, was phosphorylated in the presence of γ-[^{32}P]-ATP, Mg^{2+}, and a partly purified cyclic AMP-dependent protein kinase from beef skeletal muscle. The phosphorylation was strongly stimulated by cyclic AMP. The bulk of the membrane-attached ^{32}P-phosphate was covalently bound to protein, was resistant to hydroxylamine, which decomposes acyl phosphate, and could largely be recovered as seryl phosphate on partial acid hydrolysis.

Since membranes possessing intrinsic cyclic AMP-dependent protein kinase activity could not be isolated from pig myocardium by the Portius-Repke (Portius and Repke, 1967) method, which utilized prolonged extraction with 0.4 M LiBr, a second series of phosphorylation experiments was carried out on a vesicular pig heart preparation (Langslet and Øye, 1970) rich in cell surface membrane fragments, as indicated by enzyme marker identification, and lacking features characteristic of sarcoplasmic reticulum. This membrane preparation contained a protein kinase that could be stimulated by cyclic AMP. Fig.7 shows the time course of intrinsic protein phosphorylation in this preparation during incubation in slightly modified (Kuo and Greengard, 1970) medium containing γ-[^{32}P] ATP, i.i. the transfer of the terminal phosphate of ATP to a membrane protein by membrane-

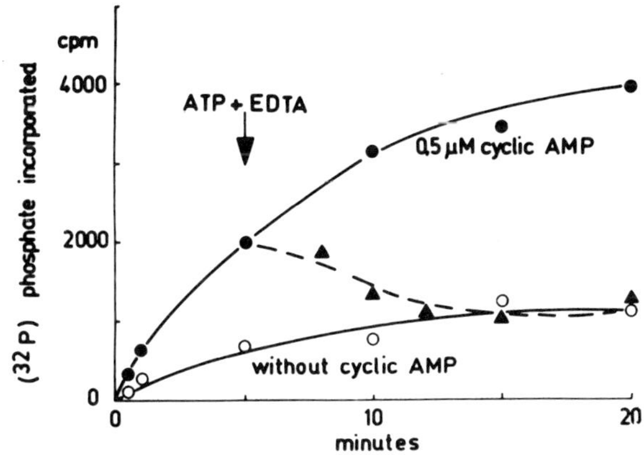

Figure 7. Protein phosphorylation and dephosphorylation in a cell membrane-enriched subcellular fraction of pig myocardium (Krause et al., 1973). At the time marked by the arrow, EDTA (final concentrationion 3.7 mM) and ATP (final concentration 0.39 mM, corresponding to a 20-fold dilution of ^{32}P-ATP, were added to the reaction mixture.

bound protein kinase. The reaction was strongly stimulated by 5×10^{-7}M cyclic AMP (Krause et al., 1973). Half-maximal stimulation was obtained at a concentration of 3×10^{-8}M. At the time marked by the arrow, unlabelled ATP and EDTA were in some experiments added to the reaction mixture to stop ^{32}P incorporation. At once ^{32}P label began to come off the membrane protein, obviously due to a dephosphorylation reaction catalyzed, as we think, by membrane-bound phosphoprotein phosphatase.

Interestingly enough, proteins which usually are good substrates for cyclic AMP-dependent protein kinases, such as histones and protamine, were not phosphorylated when added to the membrane preparation either in the absence or presence of cyclic AMP. In this respect our protein kinase differs from the cyclic AMP-dependent protein kinase in cardiac sarcoplasmic reticulum, which according to Wray et al., (1973) does phosphorylate histones. However, when our protein kinase was partly solubilized by treatment of the membrane preparation with 0.2% Triton x-100, it phosphorylated histones at a high rate, especially F_3 histone. This behaviour suggests that the enzyme may be built into the membrane in a way that makes it inaccessible to exogenous substrates, existing perhaps in a tight complex with its endogenous protein substrate.

When after the phsophorylation reaction the membrane fragments were solubilized in 3% sodium dodecyl sulfate (SDS)-mercaptoethanol solution and subjected to SDS-acrylamide electrophoresis (Krause et al., in press), about 90 per cent of the incorporated activity was present in a minor protein band migrating at a speed of a protein of a molecular weight of 24,000 daltons; the remaining 10 per cent was associated with a protein of an estimated molecular weight of about 90,000 daltons (Fig.8). The increment in bound radioactivity due to cyclic AMP was confined to the band containing the 24,000 dalton protein. No

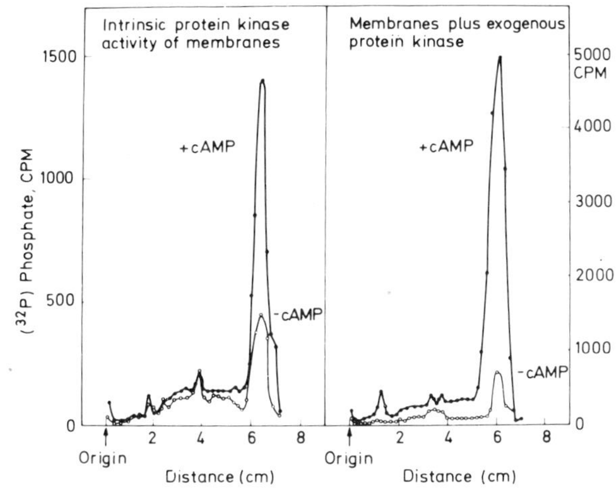

Figure 8. Resolution by SDS-acrylamide gel electrophoresis of membrane-associated substrate(s) of cyclic AMP-dependent membrane-associated and exogenous protein kinases. The cyclic AMP concentration during a 1-min incubation with γ-$[^{32}P]$ATP was 5×10^{-7}M. Following electrophoresis through 0.1% SDS-10% acrylamide the gels were stained with Comassie blue and sliced into 2 mm sections for determination of radioactivity. For further details see legend of Fig.7 and text. From Krause et al.,(in press).

additional protein in the membrane preparation was phosphorylated in the presence of a partly purified cyclic AMP-dependent protein kinase from pig heart, but ^{32}P incorporation into the 24,000 dalton protein was markedly enhanced by this kinase plus cyclic AMP (Fig.8). That the labelled phosphate transferred from the γ-[^{32}P] ATP was covalently bound to protein is suggested by the fact that it was not removed by cold and hot trichloroacetic acid and that little label was extracted by lipid solvents. The [^{32}P] phosphate-protein bond in the 24,000 dalton proteins as alkali-labile and as not split by hydroxylamine. This property and its relatively high stability in acid suggests that it is a phosphoester bond and more or less excludes the possibility that we were dealing with the phosphorylated forms of Na^+, K^+ or Ca^{2+}-stimulated ATPase, where the phosphorus is linked to an acyl group. Indeed, after partial acid hydrolysis the bulk of the protein-bound radioactive phosphate was recovered as seryl phosphate, which is a phosphorylated amino acid characteristic of products of cyclic AMP-dependent protein kinases.

(b) Cyclic AMP-Enhanced Calcium Binding

The cell membrane preparations used in our experiments do not exhibit what conventionally is termed Ca^{2+} uptake, i.e. a protracted accumulation of the ion in the presence of oxalate, one reason being perhaps that the membrane fragments in these preparations do not form firmly closed vesicles. But they are capable of binding Ca^{2+}, with and also without ATP and Mg^{2+} being present, and they possess a small number of binding sites with high affinities for the metal ion (Will et al., 1973).

The Scatchard plots (Scatchard, 1949) displayed in Fig.9

represent the results of experiments with membrane vesicles from pig myocardium prepared according to Matsui and Schwartz,(1966). They demonstrate three facts: (1) the membranes possess multiple classes of Ca^{2+} binding sites, as indicated by the curvilinearity ; (2) Ca^{2+} binding is enhanced by ATP plus Mg^{2+} ; and (3) Ca^{2+} binding, both in the absence and presence of MgATP, is enhanced by cyclic AMP-dependent protein phosphorylation. In these experiments, the incorporation of phosphate due to cyclic AMP was about 150 pmoles per mg protein. The amount of protein used for measuring binding was 0.5 mg/ml. After incubation with ^{45}Ca at 20°C, the particles were collected by centrifugation and radioactivity was measured in the pellet and supernatant, a good balance of counts being obtained in every instance.

If we take the beginning part of the two curves in Fig. 9 for Ca^{2+} binding in the absence of ATP and Mg^{2+}, for which more data were obtained than for the other two curves, and if we expand the scale on the abscissa, we see (Fig. 10) that the two curves can each be resolved into 2 straight lines which together describe the binding of Ca^{2+} to what probably constitutes 2 classes of high affinity binding sites (Will et al., 1973). It is evident that protein phosphorylation does not alter the extrapolated maximum number of binding sites - the intercepts on the abscissa are hardly moved -, but markedly increases the affinity for Ca^{2+}.

The high affinity Ca^{2+} binding was diminished in the presence of

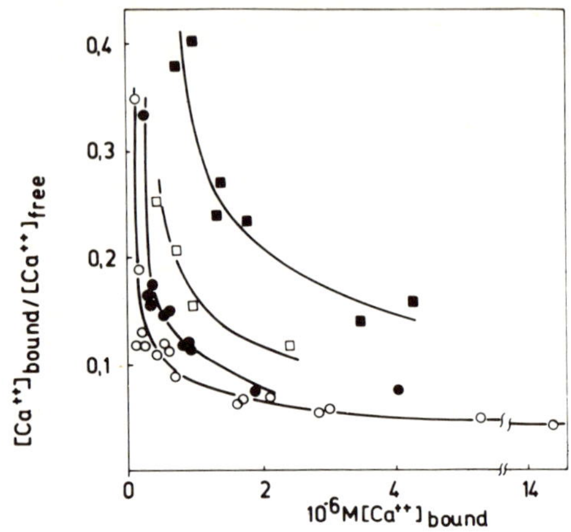

Figure 9. Binding of Ca^{2+} to cell membrane-enriched preparation from pig myocardium, expressed according to Scatchard, (1949). The membrane preparation (0.5 mg protein/ml) was incubated for 15 minutes at 20°C in the absence or in the presence of 2 mM ATP and 2 mM Mg^{2+} in 0.12 M KCl - 0.004 M Hepes-Tris buffer of pH 6.8 with varying concentrations of ionized Ca^{2+}. At free $[Ca^{2+}] < 10^{-6}M$, varying amounts of EGTA were added to obtain the desired concentration of the ion. Prior phosphorylation (see Fig. 7) was carried out for 10 min. in the presence of $5 \times 10^{-7}M$ cyclic AMP without ATP (controls) and with ATP (phosphorylated membranes). Circles : binding of Ca^{2+} without MgATP. Squares : binding of Ca^{2+} in presence of MgATP. Open symbols : controls. Filled symbols : phosphorylated membranes. From Wollenberger et al., (in press).

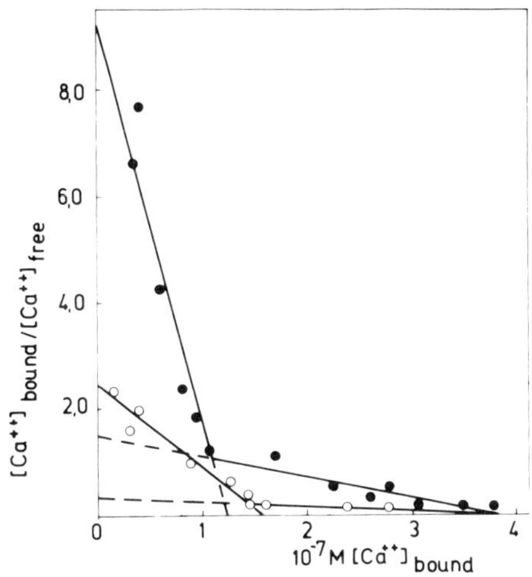

Figure 10. Scatchard plot of Ca^{2+} binding to myocardial cell membrane-enriched preparation $[Ca^{2+}]$ in absence of MgATP (Will et al., 1973).

La^{3+} and Na^{+} and by pretreatment of the membrane preparation with trypsin and phospholipase A. The latter effect suggests that a lipoprotein may be involved in the binding of Ca^{2+}. In agreement with observations made by Williamson et al.,(1973) in isolated plasma membranes from guinea pig myocardium, ruthenium red (50 μM) and verapamil (1.4 μM) were without effect on high affinity Ca^{2+} binding, but depressed low affinity binding of the ion (H. Will and B. Schirpke, unpublished). The depression by Na^{+} of Ca^{2+} binding to the high affinity Ca^{2+} sites of our

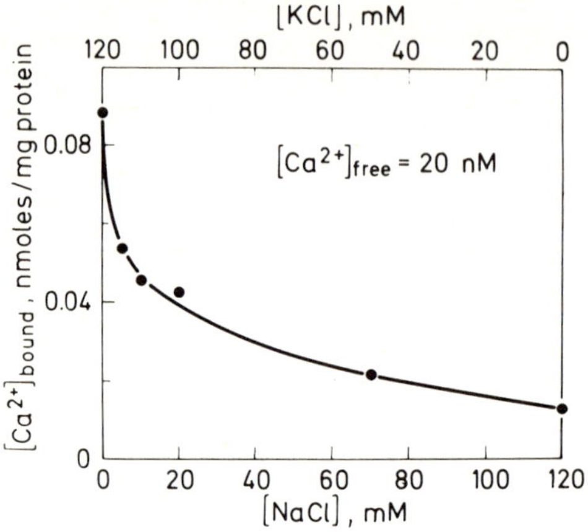

Figure 11. Inhibition of Ca^{2+} binding to cell membrane-enriched pig myocardial fraction by Na^+ (H. Will, B. Schirpke and A. Wollenberger, unpublished).

preparations is shown in Fig. 11. According to these and other data, a fifty percent inhibition of Ca^{2+} binding, at an initial free Ca^{2+} concentration in the medium of 2×10^{-8}M, is produced by 10 mM Na^+. Such marked antagonism against Ca^{2+} is not exerted by Na^+ at the Ca^{2+} binding sites of the sarcoplasmic reticulum (Palmer and Posey, 1967). Low affinity Ca^{2+} binding was not affected by Na^+.

The Ca^{2+} binding parameters for the 2 high affinity Ca^{2+} binding sites in our cell membrane-enriched pig heart preparations are listed in Table 1. As we noted before, protein phosphorylation has no effect on total Ca^{2+} binding capacity, but it causes a 4-fold increase in Ca^{2+} affinity at both sites.

The values for k_{diss} in Table 1, which represent the Ca^{2+} ion concentration at which the binding sites are half saturated with the ligand, lie in or below the range within which the Ca^{2+} concentration normally fluctuates in the myoplasm during the contraction-relaxation cycle, and are several orders of magnitude below the extracellular Ca^{2+} concentration. This fact and the small number of binding sites involved, together with the inhibition of the high affinity Ca^{2+} binding by Na^{+}, has led us to suspect (Wollenberger et al., in press), on the assumption that we were indeed dealing with properties of the cell membrane, that these sites may belong to a protein playing part in a Na^{+}-coupled extrusion process of Ca^{2+} from the cell, such as a carrier operating in intra - extracellular Ca^{2+}-Na^{+} exchange (Reuter, 1973) or Na^{+}, K^{+}-ATPase functioning as a Ca^{2+} pump, as proposed by Schon et al.,(1972). In the meantime the latter possibility has been eliminated after it was found (H. Will and B. Schirpke, unpublished) that further purification of the Matsui-Schwartz vesicles to yield a preparation of much higher specific Na^{+}, K^{+}-ATPase activity (Pitts et al., 1973) caused a loss of the high affinity Ca^{2+} binding sites. At any rate, a facilitation of Ca^{2+} outward transport by cyclic AMP-enhanced cell membrane protein phosphorylation could be a factor contributing to the relaxation-enhancing effect of the catecholamines on the heart. One can also speculate that phosphorylation of a cell membrane protein might be instrumental in opening Ca^{2+} ion channels in this membrane or in widening existing ones, thus permitting more Ca^{2+} ions to enter the myocardial fibre during membrane depolarization, as actually happens in heart muscle exposed to positive inotropic concentrations of adrenaline (Grossman and Furchgott, 1964) (Reuter, 1965) and dibutyryl cyclic AMP (Meinertz et al., 1973).

Epilogue

Fig.12 is intended to summarize the present state of our knowledge, or rather ignorance, about the relationship between protein kinase activation initiated by catecholamines and effected through cyclic AMP and the function of a number of Ca^{2+}-regulated and Ca^{2+}-regulating proteins and organelles in the myocardial cell. As pointed out earlier in this presentation, the effect of phosphorylation on the activation of phosphorylase kinase by Ca^{2+} ions (box on the far left) seems well established. Nobody has looked yet at protein phosphorylation in mitochondria (box to the far right) in relation to their Ca^{2+}-sequestring and releasing ability, although cyclic AMP has been shown to induce Ca^{2+} efflux from heart and other mitochondria (Borle, 1973). Question marks have been placed in the figure at the arrows connecting the catalytic subunit of protein kinase with the myofibrils, the sub-

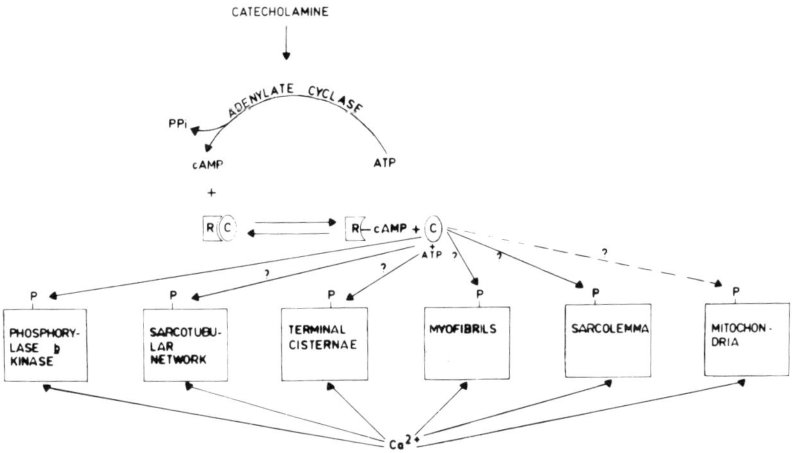

Figure 12. Possible relationship between the cyclic AMP-protein kinase system and various Ca^{2+}-regulated or regulating systems in the myocardial fiber.

structures of the sarcoplasmic reticulum, and the sarcolemma, because in addition to doubts raised about the purity of cardiac sarcoplasmic reticulum and sarcolemmal preparations obtainable by present methods, it remains to be established that the reported effects of cyclic AMP on protein phosphorylation in isolated myofibrillar and cardiac membrane preparations are not purely *in vitro* phenomena. Future work can be expected to reveal, whether such effects actually occur in the intact myocardial fiber and whether they are associated there with other biochemical and with functional changes characteristic of the action of

TABLE 1. Parameters of High Affinity Ca^{2+} Binding Sites in Cell Membrane-enriched Preparation from Pig Heart

MgATP absent. Prior phosphorylation of membranes for 10 min in presence of 5×10^{-7} M cyclic AMP, with ATP omitted in the control run (-).

From Will et al.,(1973).

Site	Phosphorylation	n, µmoles/g protein	K_{ass}, M^{-1}	K_{diss}, M
First	-	0.32	1.56×10^{7}	6.4×10^{-8}
	+	0.29	6.25×10^{7}	1.6×10^{-8}
Second	-	0.77	9.10×10^{5}	1.1×10^{-6}
	+	0.77	3.85×10^{6}	2.6×10^{-7}

substances like the catecholamines which raise in the myocardium the cellular level of cyclic AMP.

Acknowledgements

I thank Dr. E.G. Krause and Dr. H. Will for their collaboration in some of the work discussed in this presentation and for their consent to refer to unpublished data. I am also most grateful to Dr.

J.R. Williamson for kindly having given me a copy of the manuscript of his superb review on the effects of adrenaline on glycogenolysis and myocardial contractility (Williamson, in press) prior to publication.

REFERENCES

Ahren, K., Hjalmarson, Å., and Isaksson, O. (1971). Inotropic and metabolic effects of dibutyryl cyclic adenosine 3', 5'-monophosphate in the perfused rat heart. Acta physiol. scand. 82, 79-90.

Bailey, C.,and Villar-Palasi, C. (1971). Cyclic AMP dependent phosphorylation of troponin. Fed. Proc. 30, 1147.

Baudouin-Legros, M., and Meyer, P. (1973). Effects of angiotensin, catecholamines and cyclic AMP on calcium storage in aortic microsomes. Brit. J. Pharmacol. 47, 377-385.

Benfey, B.G. (1971). Lack of relationship between myocardial cyclic AMP concentrations and inotropic effects of sympathomimotic amines. Brit. J. Pharmacol. 43, 757-763.

Bertelli, A., Bianchi, C., and Beani, L. (1972). Effects of AMP and cyclic AMP on the mechanical and electrical activity of isolated mammalian atria. Eur. J. Pharmacol. 82, 130-133.

Bilezikian, J.P., and Aurbach, G.D. (1973). A β-adrenergic receptor of the turkey erythrocyte I. Binding of catecholamine and relationship to adenylate cyclase activity. J. Biol. Chem. 248, 5575-5583.

Birnbaumer, L., Pohl, S.L., Michiel, H., Kraus, J., and Rodbell, M. (1970). The actions of hormones on the adenyl cyclase system; in Greengard and Costa role of cyclic AMP in cell function, pp. 185-208. Raven Press, New York.

Boder, G.B., and Johnson, I.S. (1972). Comparative effects of some cardioactive agents on automaticity of cultured heart cells. J. Mol. Cell. Cardiol. 4, 453-464.

Borle, A.B. (1973). Cyclic AMP regulation of calcium efflux from liver, kidney and heart mitochondria. IRCS Internat. Res. Commun. Syst. (73-8) 1-3-1, 9.

Brooker, G. (1971). High pressure anion exchange chromatographic measurement of cyclic adenosine 3', 5'-monophosphate and cyclic [^{14}C] adenosine monophosphate specific activity in myocardium prelabeled with [^{14}C] adenosine. J. Biol. Chem. 246, 7810-7816.

Brooker, G. (1973). Oscillation of cyclic adenosine monophosphate concentration during the myocardial contraction cycle. Science 182, 933-934.

Brostrom, C.O., Hunkeler, F.L., and Krebs, E.G. (1971). The regulation of skeletal muscle phosphorylase kinase by Ca^{2+}. J. Biol. Chem. 246, 1061-1067.

Brostrom, M.A., Reimann, E.M., Walsh, D.A. and Krebs, E.G. (1970). A cyclic 3', 5'-AMP-stimulated protein kinase from cardiac muscle. Adv. Enzyme Reg. 8, 191-203.

Campbell, M.T., and Oliver, I.T. (1972). 3': 5'-Cyclic nucleotide phosphodiesterase in rat tissues. Eur. J. Biochem. 28, 30-37.

Cheung, W.Y., and Williamson, J.R. (1965). Kinetics of cyclic adenosine monophosphate changes in rat heart following epinephrine administration. Nature 207, 979-981.

Chiba, S., Kubota, K., and Hashimoto, K. (1972). Absence of chronotropic effects of dibutyryl cyclic adenosine 3', 5'-monophosphate on the dog S-A node. Tohoku J. Exp. Med. 107, 103-105.

Christian, D.R., Kilsheimer, G.S., Pettet, G., Paradise, R., and Ashmore, J. (1969). Regulation of lipolysis in cardiac muscle: A system similar to the hormone-sensitive lipase of adipose tissue. Adv. Enzyme Regul. 7, 71-82.

Crass, M.F. III: (1973). Heart triglyceride and glycogen metabolism : Effects of catecholamines, dibutyryl cyclic AMP, theophylline, and fatty acids. Recent Adv. Stud. Cardiac Struct. Metab. 3, 275-290.

Cutiletta, A.F., Lin, C.Y., Thilenius, O.G., and Arcilla, R.A. (1973). Effect of dibutyryl cyclic AMP on myocardial performance *in vivo*. Recent Adv. Stud. Cardiac Struct. Metab. 3, 251-259.

Danilo, P., LeBarhis, E., and Rosen, M. (1972). Effects of dibutyryl 3', 5'-cyclic AMP on electrophysiologic properties of canine Purkinje fibers. Abstr. Volunt. Papers 5th Internat. Congr. Pharmacol. p.51. San Francisco.

Danilo, P., Vulliemoz, Y., Verosky, M., and Rosen, M.R. (1973). Activation of cardiac Purkinje fiber adenyl cyclase by B-adrenergic amines. Fed. Proceed. 32, 773 Abs.

Dhalla, N.S., Chernecki, W., Gandhi, S.S., McNamara, D.B., and Naimark, A. (1973). Cardiac and metabolic effects of dibutyryl cyclic AMP in the intact dog heart and the isolated perfused rat heart. Recent Adv. Stud. Cardiac Struct. Metab. 3, 233-250.

Drummond, G., and Duncan, L. (1970). Adenyl cyclase in cardiac tissue. J. Biol. Chem. 245, 976-983.

Drummond, G.I., Duncan, L., and Hertzman, E. (1966). Effect of epinephrine on phosphorylase b kinase in perfused rat hearts. J. Biol. Chem. 241, 5899-5903.

Drummond, G.I., and Hemmings, S.J. (1972). Inotropic and chronotropic effects of dibutyryl cyclic AMP. Adv. Cyclic Nucleotide Res. 1, 307-316.

Drummond, G.I., and Hemmings, S.J. (1973). Role of adenylate cyclase-cyclic AMP in cardiac actions of adrenergic amines. Recent Adv. Stud. Cardiac Struct. Metab. 3, 213-222.

Drummond, G.I., Valadares, J.R.E., and Duncan, L. (1964). Effect of epinephrine on contractile tension and phosphorylase activation in rat and dog hearts. Proc. Soc. Exp. Biol. Med. 117, 307-309.

Ebashi, S. (1969). Ca ions as a basis of pharmacological action. In Proc. Fourth Internat. Congr. Pharmacol. (R. Eigenmann, ed) Schwabe Publ. pp. 32-54.

Ebashi, S., and Endo, M. (1968). Calcium ion and muscle contraction. Progr. Biophys. Molec. Biol. 18, 123-183.

Entman, M.L., Levey, G.S., and Epstein, S.E. (1969). Mechanism of action of epinephrine and glucagon on the heart: evidence of a cyclic 3', 5'-AMP mediated increase in cardiac sarcotubular calcium stores. Circ. Res. 25, 429-438.

Epstein, S.E., Levey, G.S., and Skelton, C.L. (1971). Adenyl cyclase and cyclic AMP. Biochemical links in the regulation of myocardial contractility. Circulation 43, 437-450.

Fleckenstein, A. Interaction of B-adrenergic catecholamines with Ca^{2+} in myocardial contraction and relaxation. In Contraction and relaxation of the myocardium (W.G. Nayler, ed). Academic Press, London, in press (this volume).

Gartner, S.L., and Vahovny, G.V. (1972). Effects of epinephrine and cyclic 3', 5'-AMP on perfused rat hearts. Amer. J. Physiol. 222, 1121-1124.

Gillibrand, I.M., and Wyse, R. (1971). Uptake of calcium ions and the β-adrenergic receptor site in cardiac muscle. Biochem. J. 125, 105P-106P.

Goren, E.N., and Rosen, O.M. (1972). Inhibition of a cyclic nucleotide phosphodiesterase from beef heart by catecholamines and related compounds. Molec. Pharmacol. 8, 380-384.

Govier, W.C. (1968). Myocardial alpha adrenergic receptors and their role in the production of a positive inotropic effect by sympathomimetic agents. J. Pharmacol. exp. Ther. 159, 82-90.

Greengard, P., and Kuo, J.F. (1970). On the mechanism of action of cyclic AMP; in Greengard and Costa Role of cyclic AMP in cell function, pp. 287-306. Ravens Press, New York.

Grossman, A., and Furchgott, R. (1964). Effects of various drugs on calcium exchange in the isolated guinea pig left auricle. J. Pharmacol. exp. Ther. 145, 162-172.

Haas, H., and Gokel, M. (1970). Der EinfluB von Verapamil auf den Myokardstoffwechsel. Arzneimittelforsch. 20, 647-655.

Haugaard, N., and Hess, M.E. (1965). Actions of autonomic drugs on phosphorylase activity and function. Pharmacol. Rev. 17, 27-69.

Haugaard, N., Levin, R.M., and Haugaard, E.S. (1973). The roles of energy sources and ions in the regulation of cardiac function. Recent Adv. Stud. Cardiac Struct. Metab. 3, 223-232.

Hechter, O. (1971). Cyclic AMP as 'second messenger': In retrospect and in prospect. Abstr. Int. Conf. Physiology and Pharmacology of Cyclic AMP, pp. 27-29. Milan.

Heilmeyer, L.M.G., and Pratje, E. (1973). The effect of phosphorylation of actin and troponin on the actomyosin ATPase. Abstr. 9th. Intern. Congr. Biochem. p 69. Stockholm.

Henion, W.F., Sutherland, E.W., and Pasternak, T. (1967). Effects of derivatives of adenosine 3', 5'-phosphate on liver slices and intact animals. Biochim. Biophys. Acta 148, 106-113.

Hess, M., and Haugaard, N. (1958). The effect of epinephrine and aminophylline on the phosphorylase activity of perfused contracting heart muscle. J. Pharmacol. exp. Ther. 122, 169-175.

Himms-Hagen, J. (1972). Effects of catecholamines on metabolism. In Catecholamines, Handbuch der Experimentellen Pharmakologie (H. Blaschko and E. Muscholl, eds) pp. 363-462. Springer-Verlag, Heidelberg.

Hutunnen, J.K., and Steinberg, D. (1971). Activation and phosphorylation of purified adipose tissue hormone-sensitive lipase by cyclic AMP-dependent protein kinase. Biochim. Biophys. Acta 239, 411-427.

Katz, A.M., and Repke, D.I. (1973). Calcium-membrane interaction in the myocardium: effects of ouabain, epinephrine and 3', 5'-cyclic adenosine monophosphate. Amer. J. Cardiol. 31, 193-201.

Katz, A.M., Tada, M., Repke, D.I., and Kirchberger, M.A. (1974). Adenylate cyclase; Its probable localization in the sarcoplasmic reticulum as well as sarcolemma of the canine heart. J. Mol. Cell. Cardiol. 6, 73-87.

Kaukel, E., and Hilz, H. (1972). Permeation of dibutyryl cAMP into HeLa cells and its conversion to monobutyryl cAMP. Biochem. Biophys. Res. Commun. 46, 1011-1018.

Kjekshus, J.K., Henry, P.D., and Sobel, B.E. (1971). Activation of phosphorylase by cyclic AMP without augmentation of contractility in the perfused guinea pig heart. Circ. Res. 29, 468-478.

Kirchberger, M.A., Tada, M., Repke, D.I., and Katz, A.M. (1972). Cyclic adenosine 3', 5'-monophosphate-dependent protein kinase stimulation of calcium uptake by canine cardiac microsomes. J. Mol. Cell. Cardiol. 4, 673-680.

Kobayashi, T., Nakayama, R., and Kimura, U. (1971). Effects of glucagon, prostaglandin E_1 and dibutyryl cyclic 3', 5'-AMP upon the transmembrane action potential of guinea pig ventricular fiber and myocardial contractile force. Jap. Circul. J. 35, 807-819.

Kono, T., and Colowick, S.O. (1961). Isolation of skeletal muscle cell membrane and some of its properties. Arch. Biochim. Biophys. 93, 520-533.

Krause, E.G., Halle, W., Kallabis, E., and Wollenberger, A. (1970). Positive chronotropic response of cultured isolated rat heart cells to N^6-2-0-dibutyryl-3', 5'-adenosine monophosphate. J. Mol. Cell. Cardiol. 1, 1-10.

Krause, E.G., Will, H., Pelouch, V., and Wollenberger, A. (1973). Cyclic AMP-dependent protein kinase activity in a cell membrane-enriched subcellular fraction of pig myocardium. Acta Biol. Med. German. 31, K37-43.

Krause, E.G., Will, H., Schirpke, B., and Wollenberger, A. (in press). Cyclic AMP-enhanced protein phosphorylation and calcium binding in a cell membrane-enriched preparation from pig myocardium. Adv. Cyclic Nucleotide Res.

Krebs, E.J., Huston, R.H., and Hunkeler, F.L. (1968). Properties of phosphorylase kinase and its control in skeletal muscle. Adv. Enzyme Reg. 6, 245-255.

Kukovetz, W.R., and Pöch, G. (1970). Cardiostimulatory effects of cyclic 3', 5'-adenosine monophosphate and its acylated derivatives. Arch. Pharmakol. 266, 236-254.

Kukovetz, W.R., and Pöch, G. (1972). The positive inotropic effect of cyclic AMP. In: Adv. Cyclic Nucleotide Res. 1, 261-290.

Kukovetz, W.R., Pöch, G., and Wurm, A. (1973). Effect of catecholamines, histamine and oxytedrine on isotonic contraction and cyclic AMP in the guinea pig heart. Arch. Pharmacol. 278, 403-424.

Kuo, J.F., and Greengard, P. (1970). Cyclic nucleotide-dependent protein kinases. VI Isolation and partial purification of a protein kinase activated by guanosine 3', 5'-monophosphate. J. Biol. Chem. 245, 2493-2498.

Langer, G.A. (1971). Coupling calcium in mammalian ventricle: its course and factors regulating its quantity. Cardiovasc. Res. Suppl. 1, 71-75.

Langer, G.A. (1973). Heart: Excitation-contraction coupling. Ann. Rev. Physiol. 35, 55-86.

Langslet, A., and Øye, I. (1970). The role of cyclic 3', 5'-AMP in the cardiac response to adrenaline. Europ. J. Pharmacol. 12, 137-144.

La Raia, P.J., Zwerling, L.J., and Morkin, E. (1973). Phosphorylation-dephosphorylation of cardiac microsomes: A possible mechanism for control of calcium uptake by cyclic-AMP. Fed. Proceed. 32, 346.

Matsui, H., and Schwartz, A. (1966). Purification and properties of a highly active, ouabain sensitive Na^+, K^+-dependent adenosinetriphosphatase from cardiac tissue. Biochim. Biophys. Acta 128, 380-390.

Mayer, S.E. (1970). Adrenergic receptors for metabolic responses in the heart. Fed. Proc. 29, 1367-1372.

Mayer, S.E., Cotten, M. de V., and Moran, N.C. (1963). Dissociation of the augmentation of cardiac contractile force from the activation of myocardial phosphorylase by catecholamines. J. Pharmacol. Exp. Ther. 139, 275-282.

McNaughton, P.A., and Noble, D. (1973). The role of intracellular calcium ion concentration in mediating the adrenaline-induced acceleration of the cardiac pacemaker potential. J. Physio. 224, 53P-54P.

McNeill, J.H., Davis, R.S., and Muschek, L.D. (1972). Phenylephrine effects on cardiac contractility, adenyl cyclase, and phosphorylase. Arch. Internat. Pharmacodyn. Ther. 197, 317-327.

McNeill, J., and Verma, S.C. (1973). Phenylephrine-induced increases in cardiac contractility, cyclic adenosine monophosphate and phosphorylase a. J. Pharmacol. Exp. Ther. 187, 296-299.

Meinertz, T., Nawrath, H., and Scholz, H. (1972). Uber die positiv inotrope Wirkung von Dibutyryl-3', 5'-AMP an isolierten Rattenvorhöfen. Pflügers Arch. Res. Physiol. 333, 197-212.

Meinertz, T., Nawrath, H., and Scholz, H. (1973). Influence of cyclization and acyl substitution on the inotropic effects of adenine nucleotides. Arch. Pharmacol. 278, 165-178.

Meinertz, T., Nawrath, H., and Scholz, H. (1973). Stimulatory effects of DB-c-AMP and adrenaline on myocardial contraction and ^{45}Ca exchange. Experiments at reduced calcium concentration and low frequencies of stimulation. Arch. Pharmacol. 279, 327-338.

Morad, M., and Rellet, E.L. (1972). Relaxing effects of catecholamines on mammalian heart. J. Physiol. 224, 537-558.

Namm, D.H., and Mayer, S.E. (1968). Effects of epinephrine on cardiac cyclic 3', 5'-AMP, phosphorylase kinase, and phosphorylase. Molec. Pharmacol. 4, 61-69.

Nayler, W.G. (1967). Calcium exchange in cardiac muscle. A basic mechanism of drug action. Amer. Heart J. 73, 379-394.

Opie, L.H. (1968). Metabolism of the heart in health and disease. Part 1. Amer. Heart J. 76, 685-698.

Øye, I. (1965). The mode of action of adrenaline in the isolated rat heart (Universitätsforlaget, Oslo).

Øye, I., and Langslet, A. (1972). The role of cyclic AMP in the inotropic response to isoprenaline and glucagon. Adv. Cyclic Nuelcotide Res. 1, 291-300.

Øye, I., and Osnes, J.B. (1973). Cyclic AMP metabolism in the perfused rat heart after different adrenergic agents. Thes. 3. Gemtag. Deutsch. Ges. Exp. Med. Berlin, DDR, pp. 40-41.

Palmer, R.F., and Posey, U.A. (1967). Ion effects on Ca^{2+} accumulation by cardiac sarcoplasmic reticulum. J. Gen. Physiol. 50, 2085-2095.

Perry, S.L. The contractile and regulatory proteins of the myocardium. In: W.G. Nayler, Ed. Contraction and Relaxation of the myocardium. Academic Press, London, in press (this volume).

Perry, S.L., and Cole, H.A. (1973). Phosphorylation of the '37000 component' of the troponin complex (troponin-T). Biochem. J. 136, 425-428.

Pitts, B.J.R., Lane, L.K., and Schwartz, A. (1973). Nature of the transport ATPase-digitalis complex: VI. Purification of and ouabain binding to a highly active Na^+, K^+-ATPase. Biochem. Biophys. Res. Commun. 53, 1060-1066.

Portius, H.J., und Repke, K.R.H. (1967). Eigenschaften und Funktion des Na^{+} + K^{+}-aktivierten, Mg^{++}-abhängigen Adenosintriphosphat Phosphohydrolase-Systems des Herzmuskels. Acta biol. med. germ. 19, 907-038.

Pratje, E., and Heilmeyer, L.M.G. (1972). Phosphorylation of rabbit muscle troponin and actin by a 3', 5'-c-AMP-dependent protein kinase. FEBS letters 27, 89-93.

Rasmussen, H. (1970). Cell communication, calcium ion, and cyclic adenosine monophosphate. Science 170, 404-412.

Rasmussen, H., and Tennenhouse, A. (1968). Cyclic adenosine monophosphate, Ca^{++}, and membranes. Proc. Nat. Acad. Sci. Wash. 59, 1364-1370.

Rebhuhn, L.I., and Villar-Palasi, C. (1973). Stimulation of purified muscle protein kinase by cyclic AMP and its butyrated derivatives. Biochim. Biophys. Acta 321, 165-170.

Reddy, Y.S., Ballard, D., Giri, N.Y., and Schwartz, A. (1973). Phosphorylation of cardiac native tropomyosin and troponin: Inhibitory effect of actomyosin and possible presence of endogenous myofibrillar-located cyclic AMP-dependent protein kinase. J. Mol. Cell. Cardiol. 5, 461-471.

Reiter, M. (1972). Differences in the inotropic cardiac effects of noradrenaline and dihydro-ouabain. Arch. Pharmacol. 275, 243-250.

Reuter, H. (1965). Über die Wirkung von Adrenalin auf den cellulären Ca-Umsatz des Meerschweinchenvorhofs. Arch. Exp. Pathol. Pharmakol. 251, 401-412.

Reuter, H. (1973). Divalent cations as charge carriers in excitable tissues. Progr. Biophys. Mol. Biol. 26, 1-13.

Robison, G.A., Butcher, R.W., Oye, I., Morgan, H.E., and Sutherland, E.W. (1965). The effect of epinephrine on adenosine-3', 5'-phosphate levels in the isolated perfused rat heart. Mol. Pharmacol. 1, 168-177.

Robison, G.A., Butcher, R.W., and Sutherland, E.W. (1971). Cyclic AMP. Academic Press, New York.

Rodnight, R., and Weller, M. (1972). The effect of cyclic AMP on membrane-bound protein kinases and phosphatases in mammalian tissues. In: B.R. Rabin and R.B. Freedman, Eds. Effects of drugs on cellular control mechanisms. McMillan Press Ltd., London, pp. 175-192.

Sabatini-Smith, S. (1971). The effects of prostaglandins E_1 and $E_2\alpha$, norepinephrine, and 3', 5'-adenosine monophosphate on calcium transport in electrically stimulated cardiac sarcoplasmic reticulum. Fed. Proc. 30, 635.

Scatchard, G. (1949). The attractions of proteins for small molecules. Ann. N.Y. Acad. Sci. 51, 660-672.

Schön, R., Schönfeld, W., Menke, K.H., and Repke, K.R.H. (1972). Mechanism and role of Na^+/Ca^{++} competition in (NaK)-ATPase. Acta Biol. Med. German. 29, 643-659.

Schramm, M., Feinstein, H., Naim, E., Lang, M., and Lasser, M. (1972). Epinephrine binding to the catecholamine receptor and activation of the adenylate cyclase in erythrocyte membranes. Proc. Nat. Acad. Sci. USA 69, 523-527.

Schulze, W., and Wollenberger, A. Cytochemical studies on sarcolemmal adenosine triphosphatases. Recent Adv. Studies Cardiac Struct. Metab. 6 (in press).

Shahab, L., Haase, M., Schiller, U., und Wollenberger, A. (1969). Noradrenalinabgabe aus dem Hundeherzen nach vorubergehender Okklusion einer Coronararterie. Acta Biol. Med. German. 22, 135-143.

Shanfeld, J., Frazer, A., and Hess, M.F. (1969). Dissociation of the increased formation of cardiac adenosine 3', 5'-monophosphate from the positive inotropic effect of norepinephrine. J. Pharmacol. Exp. Ther. 169, 315-320.

Shinebourne, E.A., Hess, M.L., White, R.J., and Hamer, J. (1969). Effect of noradrenaline on the calcium uptake of sarcoplasmic reticulum. Cardiovasc. Res. 3, 113-119.

Shinebourne, E.A., and White, R. (1970). Cyclic AMP and calcium uptake of the sarcoplasmic reticulum in relation to increased rate of relaxation under the influence of catecholamines. Cardiovasc. Res. 4, 194-200.

Skelton, C.L., Levey, G.S., and Epstein, S.E. (1970) Positive inotropic effects of dibutyryl adenosine 3', 5'-monophosphate. Circ. Res. 26, 35-43.

Soderling, T.R., Hickenbottom, J.P., Reimann, E.M., Hunkeler, F.L., Walsh, D.A., and Krebs, E.G. (1970). Inactivation of glycogen synthetase and activation of phosphorylase kinase by muscle adenosine 3', 5'-monophosphate-dependent protein kinases. J. Biol. Chem. 245, 6317-6328.

Stull, J.T., Brostrom, C.O., and Krebs, E.G. (1972). Phosphorylation of the inhibitor component of troponin by phosphorylase kinase. J. Biol. Chem. 247, 5272-5274.

Sulakhe, P.V., and Dhalla, N.S. (1970). Excitation-contraction coupling in the heart. III. Evidence against the involvement of adenosine cyclic 3', 5'-monophosphate in calcium transport by sarcotubular vesicles of canine myocardium. Molec. Pharmacol. 6, 659-666.

Sulakhe, P.V., and Dhalla, N.S. (1973). Adenylate cyclase of heart sarcotubular membranes. Biochim. Biophys. Acta, 293, 379-394.

Sutherland, E.W., Øye, I., and Butcher, R.W. (1965). The action of epinephrine and the role of the adenyl cyclase system in hormone action. Recent. Progr. Hormone Res. 21, 623-646.

Sutherland, E.W., Robison, G.A., and Butcher, R.W. (1968). Some aspects of the biological role of adenosine 3', 5'-monophosphate (cyclic AMP). Circulation 37, 279-306.

Tada, M., Finney, J.O., Swartz, M.H., and Katz, A.M. (1972). Preparation and properties of plasma membranes from guinea pig hearts. J. Mol. Cell. Cardiol. 4, 417-426.

Teo, T.S., and Wang, J.H. (1973). Mechanism of activation of a cyclic adenosine 3': 5'-monophosphate phosphodiesterase from bovine heart by calcium ions. Identification of the protein activator as a Ca^{2+} binding protein. J. Biol. Chem. 248, 5950-5955.

Tsien, R.W. (1973). Adrenaline-like effects of intracellular iontophoresis of cyclic AMP in cardiac Purkinje fibres. Nature, N.B. 245, 120-122.

Tsien, R.W., Giles, W., and Greengard, P. (1972). Cyclic AMP mediates the effect of adrenaline on cardiac Purkinje fibres. Nature New. Biol. 240, 181-183.

Tuganowski, W., Krause, M., and Korczak, K. (1973). The effect of dibutyryl 3', 5'-cyclic AMP on the cardiac pacemaker, arrested with reserpine and -methyl-tyrosine. Arch. Pharmacol. 280, 63-70.

Walsh, D.A., Perkins, J.P., and Krebs, E.G. (1968). An adenosine 3', 5'-monophosphate-dependent protein kinase from rabbit skeletal muscle. J. Biol. Chem. 243, 3763-3765.

Warbanow, W. and Wollenberger, A. (1974). Effects of dibutyryl cyclic AMP and dibutyryl cyclic GMP on the contraction of isolated rat myocardial cells cultured in vitro. Abstr. Sympos. Adaptability of cardiac muscle, Prague, p.

Wastila, W.B., Su, J.Y., Friedman, W.F., and Mayer, S.E. (1972). Blockade of biochemical and physiological responses of cardiac muscle to norepinephrine by N-tert.-butylmethoxamine (butoxamine). J. Pharmacol. Exp. Ther. 181, 126-138.

Wildenthal, K. (1973). Maturation of responsiveness to cardioactive drugs. Differential effects of acetylcholine, norepinephrine, theophylline, tyramine, glucagon, and dibutyryl cyclic AMP on atrial rate in hearts of fetal mice. J. Clin. Invest. 52, 2250-2258.

Will, H., Schirpke, B., and Wollenberger, A. (1973). Binding of calcium to a cell membrane-enriched preparation from pig myocardium: Increase in calcium affinity upon membrane protein phosphorylation enhanced by a membrane-bound cyclic AMP-dependent protein kinase. Acta Biol. Med. Germ. 31, K45-52.

Williamson, J.R. Effects of epinephrine on glycogenolysis and myocardial contractility. Handbook of Physiology, in press.

Williamson, J.R., and Scarpa, A. (1973). Characterization of plasma membrane from guinea pig heart: Preparation by zonal centrifugation. Fed. Proceed. 32, 555 Abs.

Williamson, J.R., Scarpa, A., and Woodrow, M.L. (1973). Calcium binding to isolated plasma membranes from guinea pig myocardium. Circul. 48, Suppl. IV: 26.

Williamson, J.R., and Jamieson, D. (1965). Dissociation of the inotropic from the glycogenolytic effect of epinephrine in the isolated rat heart. Nature 206, 364-367.

Wollenberger, A. (1964). Rhythmic and arrhythmic contractile activity of single myocardial cells cultured _in vitro_. Circ. Res. Suppl. 14, 15, 184-201.

Wollenberger, A., Babskii, E.B., Krause, E.G., Genz, S., Blohm, D., and Bogdanova, E.V. (1973). Cyclic changes in levels of cyclic AMP and cyclic GMP in frog myocardium during the cardiac cycle. Biochem. Biophys. Res. Commun. 55, 446-452.

Wollenberger, A., and Krause, E.G. (1973). Neurohumoral and non-humoral regulation of glycogenolysis in the ischemic myocardium. In: J. Knoll, L. Szekeres and J.G. Papp, Eds., Symposium on Drugs and Heart Metabolism, Proc. 1st Congr. Hung. Pharmacol. Soc. pp. 19-35, Akademiai Kiado, Budapest.

Wollenberger, A., and Krause, E.G. (1973). Cyclic nucleotides and the regulation of the heart beat. Proc. 5th Internat. Congr. Pharmacol. San Francisco 1972, Vol. 5 (R.A. Maxwell, Ed.) pp. 170-191, Karger Basel.

Wollenberger, A., Krause, E.G., and Heier, G. (1969). Stimulation of 3', 5'-cyclic AMP formation in dog myocardium following arrest of blood flow. Biochem. Biophys. Res. Commun. 36, 664-670.

Wollenberger, A., Schulze, W., and Krause, E.G. (1973). On the cytochemical localization of catecholamine-sensitive adenylate cyclase activity in heart muscle. In: H. Roskamm and H. Reindell, Eds., Das chronisch kranke Herz. F.K. Schattauer Verlag, Stuttgart, pp. 143-146.

Wollenberger, A., Will-Shahab, L., Krause, E.G., Genz, S., Warbanow, W., and Nitschkoff, S. (1973). Effect of acute ischemia on myocardial cyclic AMP, phosphorylase a, and lactate levels in various forms of cardiac hypertrophy. Correlation with cardiac norepinephrine stores. Recent. Adv. Stud. Cardiac Struct. Metab. 3, 551-559.

Wollenberger, A., Will, H., and Krause, E.G. Cyclic AMP, the myocardial cell membrane, and calcium. Recent Adv. Stud. Cardiac Struct. Metab. 5, in press.

Wray, H.L., Gray, R.R., and Olsson, R.A. (1973). Cyclic adenosine 3', 5'-monophosphate-stimulated protein kinase and a substrate associated with cardiac sarcoplasmic reticulum. J. Biol. Chem. 248, 1496-1498.

Sympathetic Nerves to the Heart

R. J. LINDEN

Cardiovascular Unit, University of Leeds, U.K.

SYMPATHETIC NERVES TO THE HEART

It has been known since the writings of von Bezold (1863) that the sympathetic nerves affect the heart; increased activity in sympathetic nerves causes an increase in heart rate and an increase in the force of contraction of the heart muscle.

In this chapter no comment will be made on the effect of nerves on the coronary vessels and the conducting system, disorders of which may have an important bearing on some disease processes. However, it is necessary to point out that an increased activity in parasympathetic nerves (vagi) causes a decrease in the heart rate, a depression of the force of contraction of atrial muscle (Sarnoff et al., 1960; Linden,

1963) but almost no effect on the ventricular muscle (Sarnoff et al., 1960; Furnival, Linden and Snow, 1973a), in contrast with the increased force of contraction of both atrial and ventricular muscle brought about by increased sympathetic activity.

It is important to examine the responses to an increase in sympathetic activity in many different ways so that a whole "picture" may be built which will establish the full effect. Such knowledge should allow a more reasonable interpretation to be made of the effects of increased sympathetic activity observed in the whole animal and man and again of the effects of blockade of such activity with the new adreno-receptor blocking drugs.

<u>Anatomy</u> The course of the sympathetic nerves to the heart of the dog has been described in detail (Nonidez, 1939; Mizeres, 1955, 1958) and anatomical differences exist between the nerves of the right and those of the left. On each side the ansa subclavia, arising from the stellate ganglion, comprises two limbs which loop around the subclavian artery, re-uniting close to the vago-sympathetic trunk. The limbs of the ansae subclaviae contain almost all the sympathetic nerves to the heart (Mizeres, 1958). On the right side the majority of sympathetic nerve fibres pass to the heart in the stellate cardiac nerves and many of these fibres enter the wall of the right atrium (Mizeres, 1958); on the left the stellate cardiac nerve is often

absent and the majority of fibres pass in the centro-lateral cervical cardiac nerve to reach the dorsal ventricular plexus (Mizeres, 1955).

Effects of Stimulation of Efferent Sympathetic Nerves

Most of the investigations which illustrate the function of sympathetic nerves have been completed in anaesthetized animals. In this chapter I will not attempt to be comprehensive but will cite examples of effects mainly from our work in anaesthetized dogs. Mostly, dogs were anaesthetized with chloralose, the chest opened and the two ansae subclaviae carrying all the sympathetic efferent nerves to the heart, were freed, sectioned at their junction with the stellate ganglia and placed on stimulating electrodes. Various pressures, flows and changes in volume were measured.

Stimulating the right ansa subclavia in the anaesthetized dog, with both vagi sectioned, results in an increase in heart rate, a rise in systemic arterial blood pressure, a rise in pulmonary artery pressure and a fall in right and left atrial pressures as shown in Fig. 1. This dramatic response was a result of stimulating with supramaximal pulses at 5 pulses/sec. Admittedly, the stimulus is a large one, involving all the nerve fibres in one ansa subclavia but the full range of effect is usually not observed until a frequency of stimulation of 15 pulses/sec is used.

That this effect is not just a phenomenon observed in anaesthetized

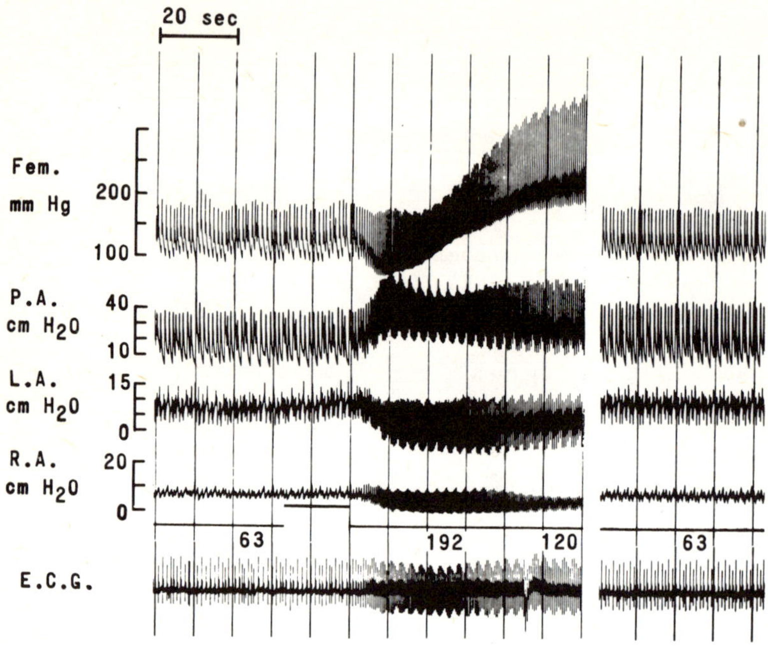

Figure 1.

Effect of stimulation of sympathetic nerves in the dog on systemic arterial blood pressure (Fem.), pulmonary artery pressure (P.A.), left atrial pressure (L.A.), right atrial pressure (R.A.) and E.C.G. Period of stimulation is indicated by upward deflection of signal and numbers on the record indicate heart rates. Both vagi and sympathetic nerves were sectioned.

animals is shown in Fig. 2, taken from Braunwald (1965). Here is shown a record from man where the left stellate ganglion was stimulated at thoracotomy. The response was an increase in systemic arterial blood

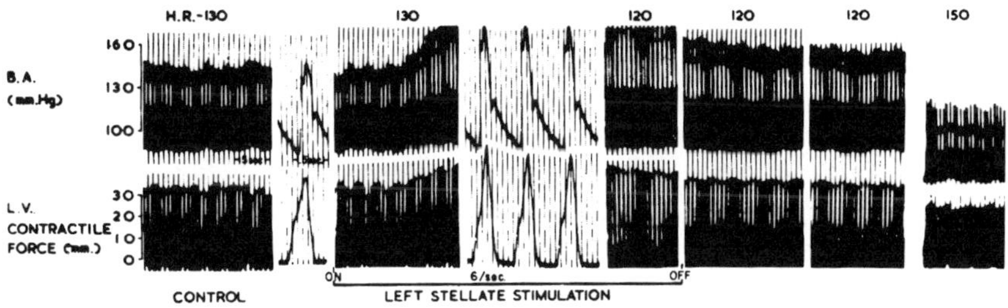

Figure 2.

Stimulation of stellate ganglion in man (period of stimulation indicated by solid bar). Numbers above record indicate heart rates. (From Braunwald, 1965).

pressure and an increase in contractile force of the left ventricle (indicated by a sewn-on strain gauge). The heart rate was a little less during stimulation, presumably because of reflex effects (baroreceptor) resulting from the increase in systemic arterial pressure; this effect is different from that observed in Fig. 1 because that record was obtained in a dog where all the nerves to the heart had been sectioned and thus no secondary reflex effects were possible. How are these effects explained?

Effects of Stimulation on Muscle of Amphibian Heart Perhaps first we could examine other experiments involving stimulation of sympathetic nerves. Gaskell collected his earlier works together in a chapter of Schafer's text book (Gaskell, 1900). Gaskell showed a beautiful record of an increase in the force of contraction of both the atrial and ventricular muscle of the toad in response to stimulation of sympathetic nerves. Both these effects observed so long ago in the amphibian have since been described in the dog; for instance, fifteen years ago Sarnoff presented elegant demonstrations of these effects in a series of reports.

Effects of Stimulation on Muscle of Dog Heart That the force of contraction of the dog atrium could be increased by increased sympathetic activity was shown by using dogs with acute and chronic heart block so that secondary ventricular effects were minimal (Sarnoff et al., 1960 ; Linden, 1963).

Again, Sarnoff, in the anaesthetized dog, paced the heart at a constant rate and stimulated the freed left stellate ganglion, and at the same time measured the arterial pressure, right and left atrial pressures and aortic flow. Reference to his Figure 1 (Sarnoff et al., 1960) shows a rise in arterial pressure, a fall in both atrial pressures and about a doubling of aortic flow during stimulation of the sympathetic nerves; presumably more blood was being transferred from the atria through the heart into the aorta. Another way of looking at this problem is to see it through the eyes of Sarnoff using his plot of "stroke work" against "end-diastolic pressure in the ventricle" or ventricular function curve (see Fig. 5 in Sarnoff et al., 1960). Here one can argue that stroke work represents the "force of contraction" and the "end-diastolic pressure" the initial fibre length - thus there is displayed a relationship according to Starling's Law. Clearly demonstrated is that the relationship changes during stimulation of sympathetic nerves - there is a "shift to the left" or at any one end-diastolic pressure in the ventricle (at any one initial length of the muscle fibre) there is a greater stroke work (greater force of contraction). There are obvious difficulties in the assumptions made - some of which are discussed by Linden (1963). Such a use of this relationship depends on the fact that the distensibility characteristics of the ventricular muscle do not change during stimulation of sympathetic nerves, a point discussed by Linden (1963).

Effect of Stimulation on Heart Volumes Another way of demonstrating the effects of sympathetic nerves on the heart is to observe the changes in the volumes of the heart. There are no very accurate methods of measuring changes in heart volume but some of Rushmer's instruments which give measurements of diameters and circumferences (see Baker et al., 1959, for references) also show changes indicating shortening of the lengths of muscle fibres during stimulation of sympathetic nerves (e.g. see Rushmer and West, 1956). However, one easy way to demonstrate changes in volumes of both ventricles is to enclose both ventricles in a cardiometer and record the changes in volume on smoked paper as described, for example, by Linden (1968). An example of such

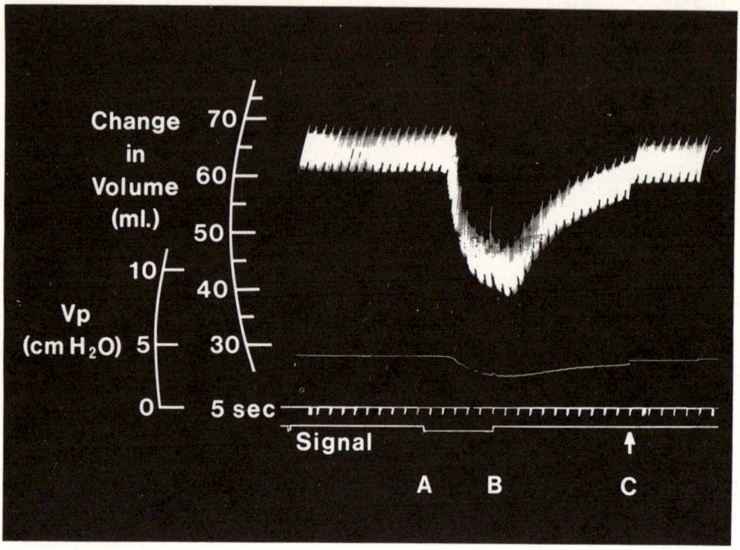

Figure 3.

Change in volume of both ventricles (indicated by cardiometer trace) on stimulation of sympathetic nerves (left ansa subclavia). Heart rate controlled by pacing, venous return constant (heart-lung preparation). Sympathetic nerves stimulated between A and B; record stopped for 1 min at C; Vp: venous pressure. (From Linden, 1968).

an experiment in a heart-lung preparation is shown in Fig.3, where the heart rate was maintained constant at 104 beats per minute and the venous inflow was constant; during the signal marker the left ansa subclavia was stimulated with supramaximal stimuli at about 4 pulses/sec (maximal responses are obtained at a frequency of stimulation of 15 pulses/sec). About 5–10 sec after the onset of stimulation (downward deflection of the signal marker) there is a decrease in the end-diastolic volume and the end-systolic volume and a fall in venous pressure (i.e. right atrial pressure). The stroke volume increases slightly at first because, even though the inflow is maintained constant, a little more blood is ejected as the heart gets smaller during the adjustment to the new smaller end-diastolic volume. Since there is little change in stroke volume and inflow is constant (because the reservoir height has not been altered) one can conclude that at least the same output has been obtained from a lower end-diastolic volume i.e. there has been a positive inotropic effect.

If now a similar experiment is done but in a dog in which the venous return is not controlled, i.e. not in a heart lung preparation, then a different response is observed. In this preparation the sympathetic nerves and the vagi are sectioned; the sympathetic nerves are then stimulated with the cardiometer in place but with no restriction on the inflow of blood to the heart. An example of a record from such an experiment is shown in Fig. 4. Here the sympathetic nerves were stimulated with supramaximal stimuli but at only 3 pulses per second and it can be seen that 4–5 seconds after the onset of the stimulation there is a decrease in the end-diastolic volume and the end-systolic volume but the end-systolic volume has decreased more than the end

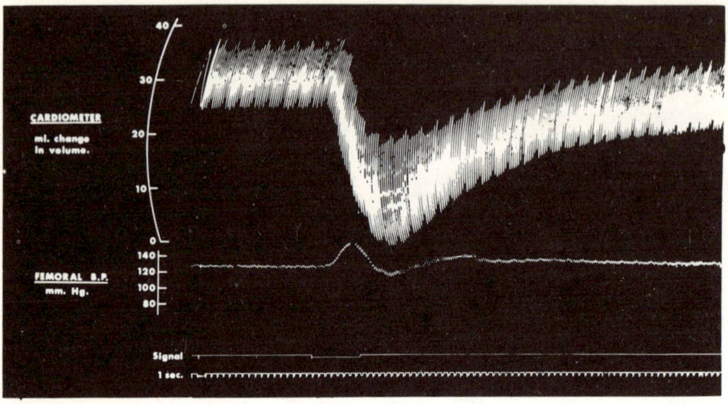

Figure 4.

Change in volume of both ventricles (indicated by cardiometer trace) on stimulation of sympathetic nerves (left ansa subclavia). Heart rate, controlled by pacing, venous return allowed to change. Sympathetic nerves stimulated during period indicated by downward deflection of signal.

diastolic volume - there is an increase in stroke volume. Because the heart was paced at a constant rate there must have been an increase in cardiac output, and the venous return must have increased as a result of the fall in right atrial pressure known to occur during sympathetic stimulation, as mentioned above.

Differential Effects of the Two Ansae Subclaviae

Having increased the information contributing to the whole

picture of the effect of stimulation of sympathetic nerves on the mechanical responses of the heart, we can now observe the effects in a little more detail.

It has been suspected since 1899 that stimulating the right ansa subclavia evoked different responses from stimulating the left (Hunt, 1899). He showed that stimulation of the left ansa subclavia resulted in an increase in blood pressure but had little effect on the heart rate, while stimulating the right ansa subclavia had a major effect on the heart rate. More recently it has been shown that stimulation of the right stellate ganglion results in a greater chronotropic but smaller inotropic response than stimulation of the left stellate ganglion (Randall and Rohse, 1956 ; Randall et al., 1968). However it is known that changes in heart rate and blood pressure have measurable secondary inotropic effects and none of these previous investigations have eliminated these secondary effects.

Primary Differential Effects In Leeds we evolved a method of measuring the changes in inotropic responses particularly to estimate the extent of secondary effects of changes in heart rate and blood pressure (Furnival, Linden and Snow, 1970). Basically the method involved recording the rate of change in pressure in the ventricle and measuring the highest value obtained during the cardiac cycle (dP/dt max; measured at the same constant paced heart rate). This measurement was shown to increase

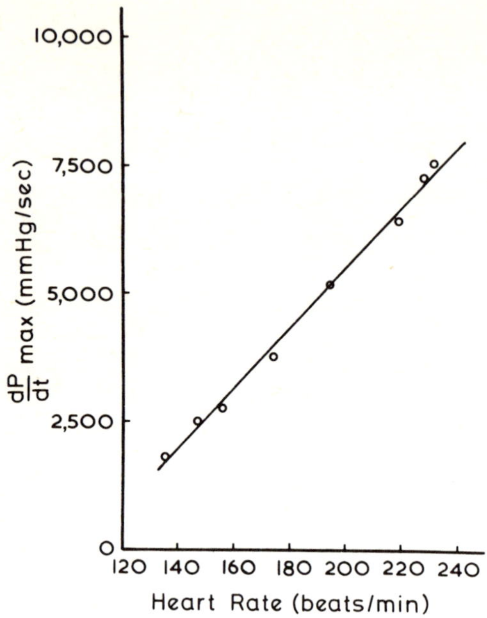

Figure 5.

The relationship between the increases in heart rate and dP/dt max brought about by stepwise infusion of isoprenaline.

with increasing infusions of isoprenaline in a manner parellel to the increase in heart rate resulting from that infusion. An example of the results obtained in one dog is shown in Fig. 5 where one response (change in dP/dt max) is plotted against the other (change in heart rate). Using this index it was shown that increases in heart rate or blood pressure caused a positive inotropic response (about 2000 mm Hg/sec per 100 beats/min increase in heart rate and about a 1000 mm Hg/sec per 100 mm Hg increase in systemic blood pressure; Furnival et al., 1970).

Thus in examining the effects of stimulating sympathetic nerves on the heart it is important to control the heart rate and blood pressure. In anaesthetized dogs we paced the heart at a constant rate and maintained systemic arterial blood pressure constant by manipulating a screw clamp on the descending aorta and/or bilateral femoral arterio-venous fistulae whilst at the same time stimulating each ansa subclavia with supramaximal stimuli at various frequencies (Furnival et al., 1973b). As an example the results from one dog are shown in Fig. 6. In this dog the heart was paced at 181 beats/min and during recording the range of mean aortic pressure was 120-130 mm Hg. Relative to the frequency of stimulation, the right ansa subclavia is associated with a greater increase in heart rate than the left ansa subclavia; while the changes in the dP/dt max show the opposite effect, the changes during stimulation on the left are greater than those during stimulation on the right. The difference between these effects is more clearly seen in Fig. 7 where the inotropic and chronotropic effects are related by showing the values of dP/dt max, at each frequency of stimulation, on the ordinate and of the simultaneous free heart rate on the abscissa. In this form the relative chronotropic and inotropic effects during stimu-

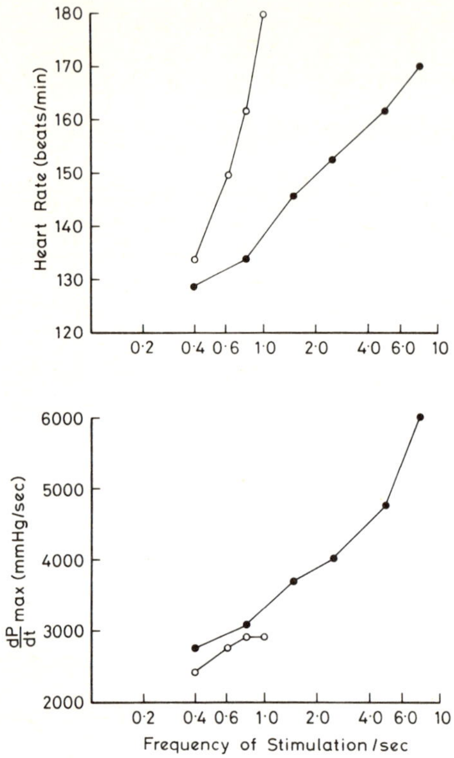

Figure 6.

Stimulus-response curves illustrating the changes in heart rate and dP/dt max in one dog, brought about by stimulating the left ansa subclavia (●) and the right ansa subclavia (o). In this experiment heart rate and blood pressure were controlled and all measurements of dP/dt max made at the same paced heart rate and mean aortic pressure. (From Furnival et al., 1973b).

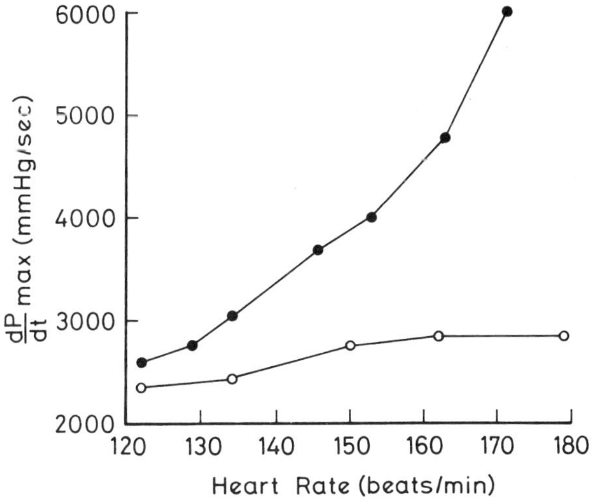

Figure 7.

The relationship between dP/dt max and heart rate in response to stimulation of the left ansa subclavia (●) and the right ansa subclavia (o). Each point represents the heart rate and dP/dt max at a particular frequency of stimulation. The values of heart rate and dP/dt max were obtained from the stimulus-response curves shown in Fig. 5. (From Furnival et al., 1973b).

lation of each ansa subclavia are expressed by the slope of the curve and may easily be compared.

The results obtained in six dogs are summarised in Table I. In this series of experiments at the same rate of stimulation, stimulation

TABLE 1

The changes in heart rate and dP/dt max produced by stimulation of the right and left ansae subclaviae. Heart rate was controlled by electrical pacing of the right atrium, and blood pressure by manipulation of a screw clamp on the descending aorta and by a femoral arteriovenous fistula. Records of control heart rate and increases in heart rate were obtained when the heart was not paced, and records of control dP/dt max and increases in dP/dt max when the heart was paced at the rate indicated. The tabulated increases in heart rate and dP/dt max were those obtained at the highest frequency of stimulation. The ratio of dP/dt max. HR^{-1} is the slope of the regression line of dP/dt max upon heart rate.

Dog No	Control heart rate (beats/min)	Increase in heart rate (beats/min)	Paced heart rate (beats/min)	Control dP/dt max (mm Hg/sec)	Increase in dP/dt max (mm Hg/sec)	dP/dt max HR^{-1}
			Stimulation of right ansa subclavia			
6	111	93	200	2484	1104	11
14	142	49	210	2015	276	6
	162	54	210	1794	414	8
66	127	62	198	2705	331	6
67	138	53	190	2070	483	9
68	122	57	181	2346	497	10
	121	62	182	2705	414	7
69	143	35	176	3175	413	19
	142	54	196	3119	1021	12
Mean	134.2	57.7	---	2490	550	9.7*
S.E. of mean	5.1	5.2	---	161	99	1.4
			Stimulation of left ansa subclavia			
6	114	28	178	2622	966	88
14	141	64	210	3058	3428	66
66	123	75	197	2981	3091	41
67	132	60	190	2070	2070	30
	138	60	195	2070	2622	38
68	115	61	181	2484	3864	60
	122	49	181	2622	3395	65
69	146	29	176	3960	6114	156
	138	26	196	3312	5658	222
Mean	129.9	50.2	---	2798	3468	84.4*
S.E. of mean	3.9	6.0	---	201	540	21.2

*The difference between the mean values of dP/dt max. HR^{-1} for the right and left ansae subclaviae is significant, $P < 0.001$, unpaired t test.

of the right ansa subclavia always resulted in a greater increase in heart rate than that which resulted from stimulation of the left ansa subclavia and conversely stimulation of the left ansa subclavia always resulted in a greater inotropic response. The range of inotropic response to stimulation of the right ansa subclavia was limited by the maximum attainable pacing rate which could be achieved without pulsus alternans and in any one dog the maximum rate of stimulation was not always as great as that used to stimulate the left ansa subclavia. There is a significant difference ($p > 0.001$ unpaired 't' test) between the mean values for the increase in dP/dt max per unit increase in heart rate brought about by stimulation of either the right or left ansa subclavia. Thus in these experiments, in which the mean aortic blood pressure and heart rate were controlled, stimulation of the left ansa subclavia results in a positive inotropic response which is about 8 times that brought about by stimulation of the right ansa subclavia, when related to the same increase in heart rate

Primary plus secondary differential effects. It is possible now to add the secondary effects of the increase in heart rate and systemic arterial blood pressure concomitant with the increase in sympathetic activity. Experiments were completed which were similar to those described above but in which the heart rate and blood pressure were allowed to change freely. The changes in heart rate and dP/dt max brought about by stimulating the

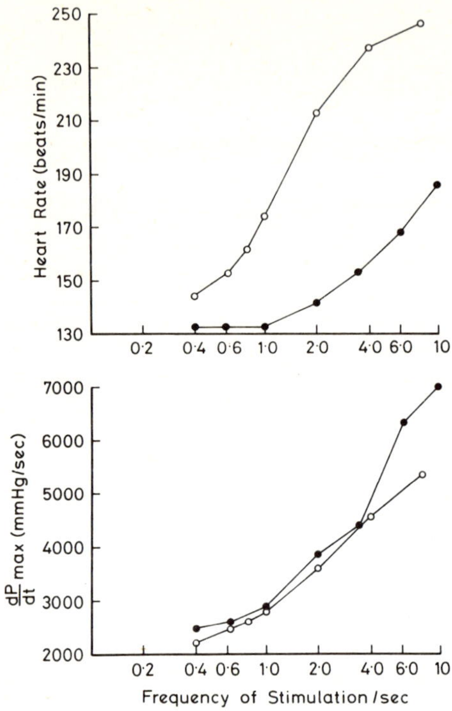

Figure 8.

Stimulus response curves illustrating the changes in heart rate and dP/dt max in one dog, brought about by stimulating the left ansa subclavia (●) and the right ansa subclavia (o). In this experiment heart rate and blood pressure were allowed to change freely. (From Furnival et al., 1973b).

right and left ansae subclaviae in one dog are shown in Fig. 8. The results show that, within the range of frequencies of stimulation used, the chronotropic and inotropic changes in response to stimulation of the two groups of nerves again are different. Again, for a given frequency of stimulation the chronotropic response when the right ansa was stimulated was greater than when the left ansa was stimulated and in this particular experiment the inotropic response was greater when the left ansa was stimulated. If the responses are plotted in a similar way to those shown in Fig. 7 in which one response is plotted against another, it can be seen that in this particular experiment (see Fig. 9) for a given increase in heart rate brought about by stimulation of the left or right ansae subclaviae, stimulation on the left side resulted in an inotropic response which again was greater than that brought about by stimulation on the right side. The relative inotropic and chronotropic effects of stimulating the two groups of nerves are expressed by the slopes of the curves as before and may easily be compared.

The results obtained in nine experiments in which the heart rate and blood pressure were allowed to change freely are summarised in Table 2. The overall mean increase in blood pressure when the right ansa subclavia was stimulated was 14 mm Hg (mean; S.E. $\pm$ 7.0) and when the left ansa was stimulated 18.2 mm Hg (mean; S.E. $\pm$ 7.0). In any one dog the maximum rate of stimulation of each ansa subclavia was not always the same but in all seven dogs, at the same rate of stimulation, stimulation of the right ansa subclavia always resulted in a greater increase in

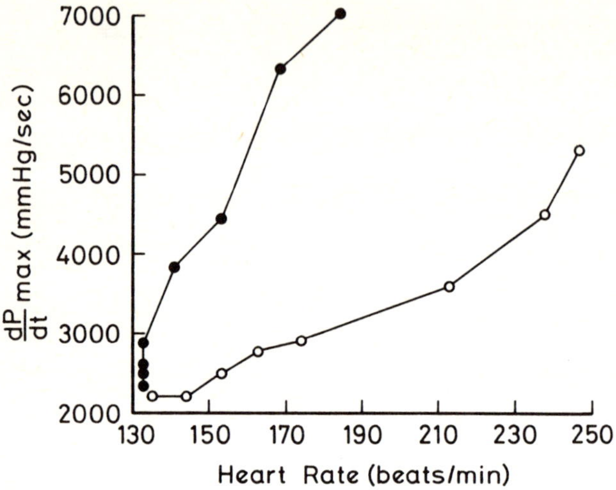

Figure 9.

The relationship between dP/dt max and heart rate in response to stimulation of the left ansa subclavia (•) and the right ansa subclavia (o). Each point represents the heart rate and dP/dt max at a particular frequency of stimulation. The values of heart rate and dP/dt max were obtained from the stimulus response curves shown in Fig. 1. (From Furnival et al., 1973b).

heart rate than stimulation of the left ansa subclavia. It can be seen from Table 2 that, comparing the slopes of the relationships between the responses as before, there is still a difference between the mean values for the increase in dP/dt max per unit increase in heart rate brought about by stimulation of the right and left ansae subclaviae and this difference

TABLE 2

The changes in heart rate produced by stimulation of the left and right ansa subclavia. Heart rate and blood pressure were allowed to change freely. The tabulated increases in heart rate and dP/dt max were those obtained at the highest frequency of stimulation. The ratio of dP/dt max. HR^{-1} is the slope of the regression line of dP/dt max upon heart rate.

Dog No.	Control heart rate (beats/min)	Increase in heart rate (beats/min)	Control dP/dt max (mm Hg/sec)	Increase in dP/dt max (mm Hg/sec)	dP/dt max. HR^{-1}
		Stimulation of right ansa subclavia			
43	152	64	4002	2346	37
45	136	135	1518	5520	41
46	136	38	1518	1380	36
48	132	129	2484	3864	30
48	135	111	2208	3174	29
49	138	66	4692	2070	31
49	138	144	3864	4692	41
52	153	96	4278	4968	52
67	138	35	2139	207	6
Mean	139.8	90.0	2967	3136	33.7*
S.E. of mean	2.5	13.9	412	594	4.2
		Stimulation of left ansa subclavia			
22	185	30	5106	3864	129
43	154	62	3864	4830	78
45	114	96	1794	6900	72
48	132	54	2346	4692	87
49	150	33	3864	3312	100
52	156	42	4002	5658	134
39	144	36	3312	6900	192
67	140	50	1932	1932	37
Mean	146.9	50.4	3278	4761	103.8*
S.E. of mean	7.3	7.6	410	610	16.8

*The difference between the mean values of dP/dt max. HR^{-1} for the right and left ansae subclaviae is significant, $P < 0.005$, unpaired *t* test.

is significant ($p > 0.005$ unpaired 't' test). However it may seem that the slope obtained by stimulating the left ansa subclavia is now only about three times that obtained by stimulating the right. Therefore the secondary effects of stimulating the right ansa subclavia have been greater than the secondary effects of stimulating the left ansa subclavia primarily because of the greater increase in heart rate and the greater secondary effect of that increase in heart rate.

Since the inotropic changes which accompany stimulation of the right ansa subclavia are relatively much less than those accompanying stimulation of the left it may be thought that the inotropic changes in the left side of the heart did not necessarily parallel inotropic changes in the right side of the heart when these changes were brought about by activity in sympathetic nerves i.e. it is possible that the right sympathetic nerves affect the right side of the heart and the left sympathetic nerves affect mainly the left side of the heart. Therefore simultaneous recordings were made of dP/dt max in both the right and left ventricles while the right and left ansae subclaviae were stimulated in turn. The results obtained during stimulation of each ansa subclavia show that the changes in the right ventricle were parallel to those previously observed in the left; the right and left sympathetic nerves affect the right and left ventricles in the same way (Furnival et al., 1973b).

In this investigation the observed difference in the dP/dt max between the controlled and the uncontrolled experiments when related to an increase in heart rate of 60 beats/min was 1440 mm Hg/sec when the right ansa subclavia was stimulated and 1164 mm Hg/sec when the left ansa was stimulated. Therefore it was possible to conclude that the greater inotropic response which occurred in the uncontrolled experiments was a direct result of the changes in the heart rate and blood pressure. More importantly it may be seen that when the right ansa subclavia was stimulated in the uncontrolled experiments the inotropic response which was secondary to the changes in blood pressure and heart rate amounted to about 70% of the total inotropic response, but when the left ansa was stimulated to about 20% of the total inotropic response; these % values may be calculated from the information presented in Tables 1 and 2. Therefore in the intact animal it may be concluded that when activity in both groups of sympathetic nerves increases the inotropic response of the heart is only partly the result of the direct effect on the muscle and that between 20 and 70% of the total of the inotropic response is secondary to changes in heart rate and mean aortic pressure.

REFLEX EFFECTS

Having shown the effects of the efferent sympathetic nerves on the heart I would like now to give examples of reflex effects mediated through the efferent pathways described above. Two examples only will be given, one emanating from receptors in the high pressure side of the circulation and one from the low pressure side. The first example is that of the arterial baroreceptors which will be reviewed only briefly because the effects of baroreceptors on the circulation have been discussed previously in this volume.

Systemic Arterial Baroreceptors

The receptors involved in this reflex are stretch receptors which have been found in the walls of the carotid sinus and the aortic arch. One problem which has been continuously investigated in this area is whether or not stimulation of the carotid sinus and aortic arch baroreceptors affects the muscle of the ventricles.

Carotid Sinus-Baroreceptors The histology of the baroreceptors in the carotid sinus and aortic arch is well known. Although the effects of carotid sinus hypotension on heart rate and vascular resistance are also well known (Heymans and Neil, 1958), there is still some uncertainty as to its effect on the inotropic state of the heart. There are several reports describing a small positive inotropic response as carotid sinus pressure is reduced, but this response was attributed by Downing and Gardner (1968) either to a concomitant fall in cerebral perfusion pressure or secondary to changes in systemic arterial blood pressure. Both inotropic and vasomotor responses are known to occur as a result of gross cerebral hypotension or hypoxaemia (Sagawa et al., 1961;

Downing et al., 1963; De Geest et al., 1965), but there is little information on the degree of cerebral hypotension or hypoxaemia required to induce responses. Thus it was not known until recently whether the carotid sinus reflex or cerebral ischaemia was of primary importance in the control of the inotropic state of the heart and of vasomotor tone.

A recent investigation (Hainsworth and Karim, 1973) has solved the problem. They determined inotropic and vasomotor responses in carefully controlled preparations in which the pressure perfusing the isolated carotid sinuses was changed while the pressure in the rostral end of the animal, perfused through the brachio-cephalic and left subclavian arteries, was held constant. They then determined the responses from changing brachiocephalic and left subclavian artery perfusion pressure but at the same time holding carotid sinus pressure constant. In some experiments they also determined the effect of arterial hypoxaemia on the responses to cerebral hypotension. They were thus able to compare, in the same animals, the responses from carotid and cerebral hypotension and to determine the circumstances in which each mechanism was likely to be important. Inotropic responses were assessed by measuring changes in the maximum rate of change of left ventricular pressure (dP/dt max) with heart rate and mean aortic pressure held constant. Vascular resistance changes were usually assessed by perfusing the descending thoracic aorta at constant flow and measuring changes in perfusion pressure. In the event they concluded that unless the arterial oxygen tension was abnormally low the carotid sinus reflex and not the cerebral hypotension was important in the control of the inotropic state of the heart and of vasomotor activity.

An example of the results of one experiment is shown in Fig. 10. It can be seen that with cerebral perfusion pressure, aortic pressure and heart rate held constant and when the carotid sinus pressure is decreased there is an increase in dP/dt max of the order of 2350 mm Hg/sec and also an increase in diastolic aortic pressure (perfusion pressure of peripheral vessels at constant flow) indicating a positive inotropic response and an increase in vascular resistance. Also in Fig. 10 it may be seen that after the left ansa subclavia had been sectioned (cutting the left sympathetic nerves to the heart) there was only a very small increase in dP/dt max (of about 200 mm Hg/sec) but there was the same increase in pressure in the descending aorta indicating that sectioning of the ansa subclavia had almost totally abolished the inotropic response but not affected the response on peripheral resistance. Hainsworth and Karim (1973) completed 37 tests in 20 dogs and observed that decreasing the carotid sinus pressure over the baroreceptor sensitivity range resulted in a 45% (18-98) increase in dP/dt max as compared with a 59% (11-219) increase in vascular resistance.

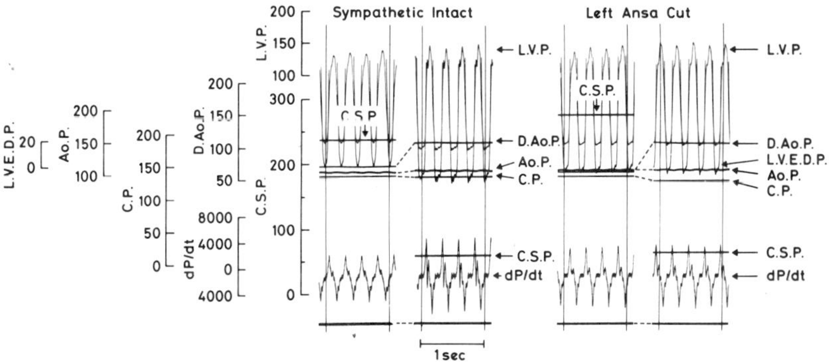

Figure 10.

Effect of reduction in carotid sinus pressure on the inotropic state of the heart before and after section of the left ansa subclavia. In this dog vasomotor responses were measured as changes in descending aortic pressure (D. Ap. P.) at constant flow. Heart paced, L.V.P., left ventricular pressure (mm Hg); L.V.E.D.P., left ventricular end-diastolic pressure (cm H_2O); C.S.P., carotid sinus pressure (mm Hg); Ao.P., aortic pressure, measured in aortic cannula (mm Hg); C.P., cerebral perfusion pressure (mm Hg); dP/dt, first differential of left ventricular pressure (mm Hg/sec). Before cutting left ansa subclavia, reducing carotid sinus pressure resulted in large increases in dP/dt max and descending aortic perfusion pressure (aortic cannula pressure, cerebral perfusion pressure and heart rate constant). After cutting left ansa, cardiac response abolished but vasomotor response persisted. (From Hainsworth and Karim, 1973).

This excellent investigation of Hainsworth and Karim (1973) as well as solving the problem of the relative importance of carotid sinus and cerebral hypoxaemia also finally settled the controversy relating to the effect of changes in activity in carotid sinus baroreceptors on the muscle of the heart - at least it is now known that lowering carotid sinus pressure causes a positive inotropic response of the left ventricle. It is interesting to note that almost all the response was abolished by sectioning the left ansa subclavia (although it must be remembered that only two dogs were investigated in this manner); as reported above, Furnival et al., (1973b) found that the left ansa subclavia contained almost all the sympathetic fibres which, when stimulated, were found to be responsible for the increased inotropic response under these controlled conditions, the right ansa subclavia having little direct effect on the heart muscle.

Aortic Arch Baroreceptors Hainsworth and Karim (1972) had previously examined the effect of aortic baroreceptors on the muscle of the left ventricle. The effect of the baroreceptors in this area had been investigated thoroughly because perfusion techniques had recently been devised which enable the aortic arch to be vascularly isolated and studies made of reflex effect of changes in aortic pressure on vascular resistance and heart rate (Daly and Daly, 1959; Daly et al., 1965 ; Levy et al., 1966 ; Hainsworth et al., 1970 ; Angell, James and Daly, 1970 ; Donald and Edis, 1971). These investigations showed that vasomotor and heart rate response from stimulation of baroreceptors in the aortic arch are qualitatively similar to those resulting from stimulation of the carotid sinus baroreceptors (Heymans and Neil, 1958). Some observations on the effects of stimulation of aortic baroreceptors on peak left ventricular pressure were made by Levy et al., (1966), but since then it has been shown that measurements of peak left ventricular pressure do not provide a sensitive or quantitative index of inotropic changes. As discussed above a much better index could be provided from measurements of the maximum rate of change of pressure in the left ventricle (dP/dt max) provided that the secondary effects of changes in heart rate and mean aortic pressure are prevented by maintaining both heart rate and mean aortic pressure constant (Furnival et al., 1970), Hainsworth and Karim (1972) perfused a pouch of the aortic arch and varied the pressure in the pouch independently of pressure in other parts of the circulation and at the same time maintained the heart rate and pressure in the ascending aorta constant while measuring the rate of change of pressure in the left ventricle.

An example of the response obtained in changing aortic pouch pressure is shown in Fig. 11 where it can be seen that lowering the pressure in the aortic pouch resulted in an increase in dP/dt max of about 3250 mm Hg/sec (aortic pressure and heart rate maintained con-

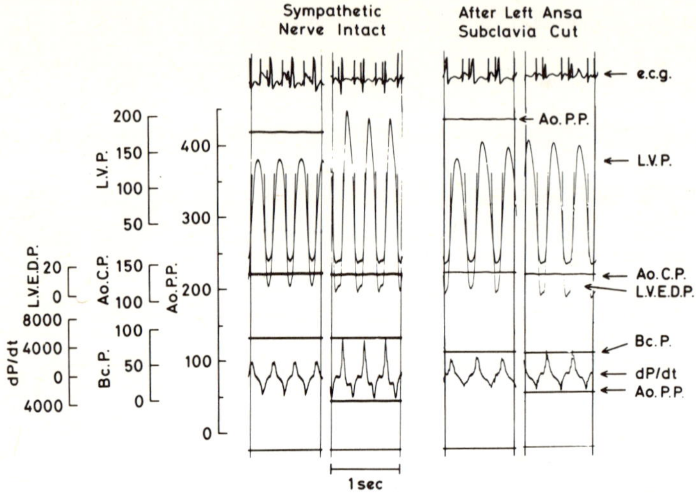

Figure 11.

The effect of a decrease in aortic pouch pressure on the inotropic state of the heart before and after section of the left ansa subclavia. Heart paced at 190 beats/min (atrio-ventricular pacing). Mean aortic cannula pressure and brachiocephalic artery pressure constant throughout. Ao. P. P., aortic pouch pressure (mm Hg); L.V.P., left ventricular pressure (mm Hg); L.V.E.D.P., left ventricular end-diastolic pressure (cm H_2O); Ao. C.P., aortic cannula pressure (mm Hg); Bc.P., brachiocephalic artery perfusion pressure (mm Hg); dP/dt, first differential of left ventricular pressure (mm Hg/sec). (Im this dog, a positive inotropic response of the heart was accompanied by a change in the E.C.G. With atrio-ventricular pacing and non-standard E.C.G. leads this is difficult to explain but it may be associated stant) which was reduced to 450 mm Hg/sec after the left ansa subclavia had been sectioned. In all, 30 tests in 12 dogs were accomplished in which a decrease in the aortic pouch pressure always resulted in an increase in dP/dt max. The average of the responses from all the dogs was an increase in dP/dt max of 1174 mm Hg/sec which represented an average increase of 43%. They also noted that after propranolol the increase in dP/dt max resulting from a large step decrease in aortic pressure was abolished or greatly reduced such that in three dogs the average response before propranolol was an increase of 1430 mm Hg/sec and, after propranolol, an increase of 40 mm Hg/sec.

It does seem therefore that we can conclude that the carotid sinus and the aortic arch baroreceptors have access to the efferent sympathetic nerves to the muscle of the heart such that decreasing the pressure in each area results in a positive inotropic response; the main efferent sympathetic pathway is possibly in the left ansa subclavia. This response is in addition to the baroreceptor effects on the heart rate also mediated partly through efferent sympathetic nerves.

---

with the changed heart size (end-diastolic pressure changes) or the rate of impulse conduction over the heart). (From Hainsworth and Karim, 1972).

REFLEX FROM ATRIAL RECEPTORS

A second example of a reflex effect on the heart mediated by efferent sympathetic nerves is that obtained by stretching the walls of the left atrium i.e. an example of a reflex from the low pressure side of the circulation. Most of the work in this field has been completed in the Cardiovascular Unit in Leeds and has recently been reviewed (Linden, 1972, 1973).

Berkley (1895) first reported a histological investigation of the sensory fibres and their end-organs in the heart. It is well known that the endocardium of both atria is the most profusely innervated, and the characteristic features of the atrial endocardium are the wealth and variety of the complex unencapsulated sensory endings found at the junctions of the superior and inferior vena cava and right atrium and of the pulmonary veins and left atrium (Linden, 1973). It was thought until recently that the endocardial atrial receptors were to be found only at the junctions of veins and atria and indeed at least two investigations (Miller and Kasahara, 1964 ; Johnston, 1968) stated emphatically that there were no receptor end-organs in the atrial appendages of dog and man, only an end net. However, Floyd, Linden and Saunders (1972) have recently given evidence that receptors are to be found in the endocardium of the atrial appendages at least of the dog and a photograph of an atrial receptor from an appendage has recently been published (Linden, 1973).

Whether stained with silver impregnation or by a supra-vital method with methylene blue the atrial receptors are observed in the loose tissue of the endocardium, all have no capsule and all appear to be stimulated by deformation of the walls of the chambers to which they are attached. An example of an atrial receptor obtained by staining with methylene blue is seen in Fig. 12. The so-called nerve net is observed throughout the atrial endocardium and an example is shown in Fig. 12; the function of this net is unknown. The examples shown in Fig. 12 were obtained in the dog but similar endings have now been observed in the cat and the monkey and Johnston (1968) has observed similar receptors in the atria of man.

Response to Stimulation of Atrial Receptors

Bainbridge (1915) observed that giving large infusions of saline or blood to the anaesthetised dog caused an increase in heart rate and Bainbridge claimed that the cause was an increased pressure in the right atrium which stimulated receptors resulting in this reflex. It is important to realise that there is no evidence in his paper from which to draw the conclusion that the right atrium had anything whatsoever to do with this reflex or combination of reflexes.

To obtain some idea of the background information and of pro-

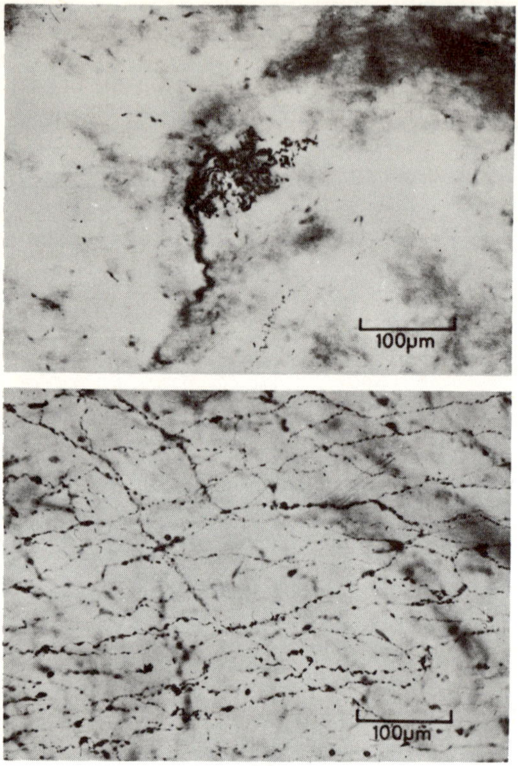

Figure 12.

Endocardium from upper pulmonary vein-left atrial junction of dog stained supravitally with a methylene blue and viewed from the surface as a whole thickness preparation. Above, one complex unencapsulated ending, a typical atrial receptor. Below, so-called nerve "net" of unknown function. (From Linden, 1973).

posed functions of atrial receptors the reader is referred to the reviews in Heymans and Neil (1958) and Paintal (1973) and to short reviews in

Ledsome and Linden (1964), Furnival, Linden and Snow (1971a), and Kappagoda, Linden and Snow (1972a).

Most of the work to be reported in the following series of experiments has been accomplished by my colleagues and me in Leeds. It was obviously an advantage to us to know exactly where the receptors were, that is, at the junctions of the veins and the atria and in both appendages. Experiments were therefore designed so that only those areas of atrio-venous wall containing atrial receptors were distended and no changes in atrial pressure or blood flow through the atria were directly caused by the distension.

It is not necessary fully to describe the experimental detail here, but it is essential to establish a few important points. First, care was taken to maintain a steady state of light anaesthesia such that there was a reflex contraction of limb muscles in response to tapping the table, and the heart rate was 10 15 beats/faster just before each 10 ml. injection of anaesthetic (chloralose) than just after. The acid-base state of the animal was kept within normal limits by altering the respiratory pump to correct P_{CO_2} changes and by giving sodium bicarbonate to correct small non-respiratory acidoses.

Left Atrial Receptors

The chest was opened in the fifth left interspace and three small balloons each about 3 mm long at the end of a short catheter, were placed one in each left pulmonary vein, so that each tip lay at the pulmonary vein-atrial junction. A soft ligature was tied around the root of the left lung immediately behind the catheter so that no blood flowed through the left lung. It was then possible to inject 0.5 - 1.0 ml. of warm saline causing each balloon to expand to a diameter of about 0.8 cm without causing any obstruction to blood flow through the lungs and atrium, and there was no rise in pressure in the atrium.

In one series of experiments action potentials or nerve impulses were recorded in slips of the vagi in the neck and then the balloons were distended. Distension of the balloons in 6 dogs caused an increased discharge in slips of the vagal nerves and we showed that the only receptors to be stimulated by the balloons were the left atrial receptors. Parts of the records from such an experiment had been published previously (Fig. 5 in Linden, 1973). We were also able to conclude from this investigation that though this balloon stimulus was so obviously "unphysiological" in one sense, it gave perfectly reasonable physiological effects in the afferent nerves from the atrial receptors - equivalent to a pressure in the left atrium of 10 - 15 cm H_2O - well within the normal physiological range. Another important observation is that though the balloon was continually distended for a period of three minutes the discharge of the receptors was pulsatile, exactly as is found if the atrium is distended in the usual way by infusing blood or saline.

Since our first investigation in 1964 (Ledsome and Linden, 1964a) in all we have now distended the small balloons in the left atrial-pulmonary vein junctions 613 times in 163 dogs and during each distension there was an increase in heart rate; the mean increase in heart rate was 25 beats/min, although the highest recorded increase in heart rate was one of 90 beats/min. There is no obvious relationship between the change in heart rate and small changes in systemic arterial pressure indicating that the carotid and aortic sinus baroreceptor mechanisms are not causing the increase in heart rate. No bradycardia has ever been observed. An example of the effect of distension of the small balloons in the pulmonary vein-atrial junctions is seen in Fig. 13, where an increase of 77 beats/min is illustrated. In Fig. 13 it is seen that the heart rate has increased from a controlled heart rate of 80 beats/min to 170 beats/min during distension of the three small balloons and is back to 105 beats/min 3 min after the distension has been removed. The increase of 77 beats/min was obtained by averaging the values of the two control periods and subtracting this value from that obtained during the distension (170 beats/min).

By sectioning and cooling the vagal nerves at various levels within the chest and in the neck it was conclusively shown that the response to distension of the pulmonary vein-atrial junctions was first reduced and then abolished by sectioning the vagal nerves. In all

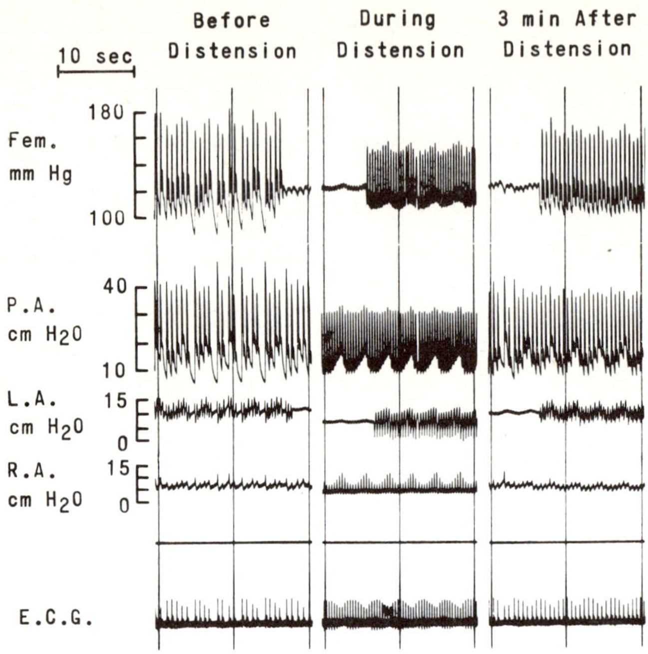

Figure 13.

Effects of stimulation of left atrial receptors on the heart rate in one dog. Parts of the femoral arterial and left atrial records show mean pressures. (From Ledsome and Linden, 1964a).

experiments it was possible to conclude that the afferent pathway was in the vagal nerves. An example of one experiment is shown in Fig. 14; here an increase in heart rate during the control distension of the pulmonary vein atrial junctions was obtained of the order of 77 beats/min but following section of the vagus nerves at the level of the right lung

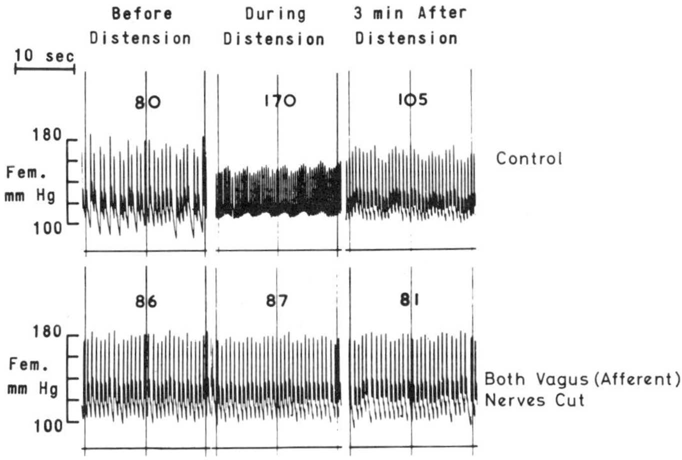

Figure 14.

Response to stimulation of left atrial receptors before and after section of both vagal nerves, right vagus at level of lung root and left at the upper border of the aorta. Numerals above records indicate heart rates.

root and the left at the level of the upper border of the aorta the increase in heart rate observed during distension of the balloons was negligible. Results similar to these were obtained from five other animals (Ledsome and Linden, 1964a).

The gradual onset and even more gradual decline of the response suggested that the efferent limb of the reflex was in the sympathetic nerves so in five dogs the effect of cutting both ansa subclaviae and

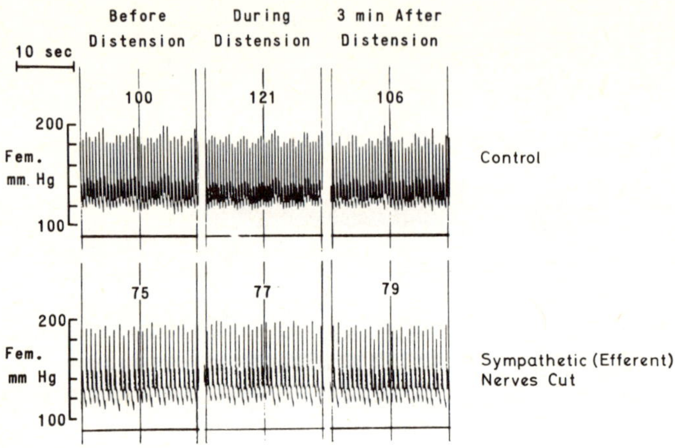

Figure 15.

Response to stimulation of left atrial receptors before and after cutting sympathetic nerves and the injection of bretylium tosylate (10 mg/kg). Numerals above records indicate heart rates.

the effect of sympathetic blockade were investigated (Ledsome and Linden, 1964a). An example of the results from one experiment in which the sympathetic nerves were blocked is shown in Fig. 15. When the atrial receptors were stimulated there was an increase in heart rate of 18 beats/min which was completely abolished by giving bretylium tosylate (10 mg/kg). Results of the five experiments show that the effects of distending the pulmonary vein-atrial junctions were produced reflexly and the efferent pathway was only in the sympathetic nerves; no vagal response was seen after full sympathetic blockade.

These results were obtained a few years ago and since then we have continuously investigated this response. In all the 613 dogs there has never been a decrease in heart rate and no evidence has been obtained that the vagal efferent nerves are involved in this reflex. In spite of this Edis, Donald and Shepherd (1970) and Burkhart and Ledsome (1974) have recently been insisting that stimulation of atrial receptors results in changes in activity in efferent vagal nerves such that increases or decreases in heart rate are observed (Edis, Donald and Shepherd, 1970) and increases in heart rate are observed (Burkhart and Ledsome, 1974).

There are several reasons for adhering to the original conclusion that the reflex which is invoked by stimulating the atrial receptors involves only a sympathetic efferent pathway and in no way involves vagal efferent nerves. First, evidence has already been produced in this chapter and in a series of publications from the Cardiovascular Unit in Leeds (see Linden, 1972, 1973 for references). All the evidence has pointed to a single sympathetic efferent pathway to this reflex. Secondly, Edis and Shepherd (1969) and Edis, Donald and Shepherd (1970) have claimed to have observed, during stimulation of atrial receptors, a reflex reduction in blood pressure and a bradycardia or a tachycardia, depending on the initial heart rate. At low heart rates a tachycardia was recorded and at high heart rates a bradycardia was recorded. No change in heart rate was observed with initial heart rates in the order of 140-150 beats/min. Their technique for stimulation of atrial receptors did not satisfy at least two primary criteria i.e. localisation of the stimulus and the ability of the stimulus to stimulate receptors under investigation; these criteria had been satisfied during the original investigation of Ledsome and Linden (1964a) where a small balloon of length 2-3 mm was distended at the vein atrial junctions and this same technique had been shown to be capable of stimulating atrial receptors to the exclusion of the other nerve endings as shown by Kidd et al., (1966).

In the preliminary communication of Edis and Shepherd (1969) three balloons each having a volume of 3-4 ml. were distended at the pulmonary vein-atrial junctions. Injection of such large volumes would undoubtedly have obstructed the flow of blood through the left atrium which has a volume of approximately 20 ml. In a subsequent paper Edis et al., (1970) described much smaller injections of saline (0.25-2 ml.) into balloons which were 1.5 cm in length. The balloons used by Ledsome and Linden (1964a) and subsequently by Kidd et al., (1966) were much smaller (approximately 2-3 mm long) and when distended with 1 ml. of saline acquired a spherical shape of diameter about 0.8 cm. While one cannot be certain of the shape acquired by a balloon 1.5 cm in length when distended with 0.25-2 ml. of saline

(Edis et al., 1970) it is unlikely either to become spherical or to stretch the vein-atrial junction in a discrete circumscribed manner. Indeed, there was no evidence to suggest that their stimulus was capable of stimulating left atrial receptors to the exclusion of other receptors. The evidence presented in their paper (Edis et al., 1970) does however support the alternative hypothesis that some of the effects noted were attributable either to obstruction to flow or to stimulation of other cardiovascular receptors. For instance distension of the balloons with 2 ml. of saline was invariably accompanied by significant diminution of cardiac output. In the presence of such changes it is clearly not possible to eliminate secondary effects of baroreceptor activity nor to attribute either the changes in heart rate or the changes in blood pressure to the stimulation of left atrial receptors alone.

Edis et al., (1970) claimed that the changes in heart rate they observed on stretching the left pulmonary vein-atrial junctions were reflexly induced. They attempted to elucidate the efferent pathway involved by the use of atropine and propranolol. The intravenous administration of propranolol did not prevent the acceleration and the administration of intravenous atropine sulphate did not prevent the slowing of the heart evoked by distension of the balloons. These two results taken individually do not provide any evidence of reflex involvement in the response. In addition, if a reflex was involved it is not the reflex increase in heart rate attributed to stimulation of atrial receptors, in which the efferent nerves are solely sympathetic, since (in the investigation of Edis et al., 1970) propranolol did not reduce the response to an increase in heart rate. It has been suggested (Furnival et al., 1971a) that at least one conclusion could be that there is no evidence of nervous involvement in the response at all.

In spite of these rather obvious shortcomings in the experiments of Edis and Shepherd, (1969) and Edis et al., (1970), Paintal (1973) has accepted the validity of the conclusion that stimulation of left atrial receptors produces a biphasic change in heart rate and a reduction in blood pressure, and proceeded to reconcile the observation from this laboratory where it has been shown that stimulation of left atrial receptors produces a consistent increase in heart rate (see above references) and small, variable and biologically insignificant changes in blood pressure. He has suggested that distension of balloons at the pulmonary vein-atrial junction produced an initial transient fall in blood pressure which is compensated by an increase in heart rate due to the activity of the baroreceptors. This contention stems from an ignorance of the nature of this transient response, which is not observed in every instance and has been thoroughly examined by Ledsome and Hainsworth (1970) and Carswell et al., (1970a). Transient responses are only observed on about 30% of the occasions on which the balloons are distended and even then there is never a bradycardia. It is apparent from all the descriptions of this reflex reported in this chapter that not even a transient bradycardia has ever been observed on distension of the pulmonary vein-left atrial junctions using the technique of the small balloons of Ledsome and Linden (1964a). There is therefore no basis for the conclusion of Edis et al., (1970) and Paintal (1973) that stimulation of atrial receptors may cause a reflex tachycardia or bradycardia, the response depending upon the initial heart rate.

Finally it is emphasized that the stimulus used by Edis et al., (1970) has not been shown to be capable of exclusively stimulating receptors and there is no evidence to indicate that flow through the left atrium was not obstructed (atrial pressures were not measured) during distension of the balloons therefore these experiments may demonstrate reflex phenomena in the circulatory system, but they shed little light on the functions of atrial receptors.

The question of obstruction to flow through the atrium even with the small balloons also occurs on reading the report of the investigation of Burkhart and Ledsome, (1974). It may be noteworthy that these investigations used smaller animals in the prone position. Again there was no measurement of left atrial pressure throughout the investigation. Burkhart and Ledsome (1974) investigated the reflex in two essential preparations, one which was decerebrate and a second which had a high spinal section in which the blood pressure was maintained by an infusion of noradrenaline. There are many criticisms of this paper but the most important one seems to stem from their records in which they examined three preparations in each of two groups. The first group of animals were decerebrate. A small increase in heart rate (6 beats/min) was observed in these animals after giving bretylium tosylate and propranolol. This increase in heart rate was not obtained following vagal section. However, after cervical vagotomy in these dogs it is noticed that even with the small balloons, distension caused a fall in blood pressure (of up to 20 mm Hg) which must have resulted from an obstruction in the left atrium and it may therefore be concluded that the obstruction was also present before cervical vagotomy possibly causing a fall in output, change in arterial baroreceptor stimulation and subsequent vagally induced increase in heart rate. Therefore, the increase in heart rate, vagally induced, is not attributable to the stimulation of atrial receptors.

In the second group, following cervical vagotomy but now after high spinal section, there were even greater falls in blood pressure (up to 60 mm Hg) when the balloons were distended. Thus, using the same argument, it is easier to explain the now greater increases in heart rate observed during distension of the balloon after high spinal section but before cervical vagotomy. It is just not possible easily to accept the conclusions from this report that the observed vagal responses are mediated through the atrial receptors.

In this regard it is difficult not to accept the evidence from this laboratory part of which is based on distension of the small balloons in the pulmonary vein-atrial junctions before and after the giving of bretylium tosylate (10 mg/kg). There is evidence that this drug blocks the effect of stimulation of sympathetic nerves to the heart and yet allows free access of afferent nerves to the efferent vagal fibers to the sino-atrial node (Ledsome and Linden 1964b). Evidence for the statement that distension of small balloons at the pulmonary vein-left atrial junctions does not cause an increase in heart rate (or any change in heart rate) following the administration of bretylium tosylate has been obtained many times in this laboratory, the first time being reported by Ledsome and Linden (1964a).

Paintal (1973) also seems to be under the impression that in Leeds we have "ignored the initial effect of distension of the small balloons" and "what Linden and his co-workers have been examining since 1964 is the effect of balloon distension on heart rate after the compensating mechanisms have come into play about 1-3 min after the start of distension." Nothing could be further from the truth. Paintal has arrived at this conclusion after mis-reading Furnival et al., (1971a) and noting only the means by which the records are reported i.e. heart rates counted 2-3 min after inflation. The records from which the heart rate counts are completed in our investigations of atrial receptors are obtained always by continuous recording. There are few transient responses and in about 70% of distensions, <u>only</u> the increase in heart rate is observed, not even a transient response. The transient response does effect blood pressure as reported by Ledsome and Hainsworth (1970) but they also pointed out that even in these dogs "the presence or absence of a fall in arterial pressure made no difference to the steady state heart rate response" and the transient changes were not affected by propranolol whereas the steady state increases in heart rates were.

There is no way in which the increase in heart rate from stimulation of atrial receptors could result from "compensation" (Paintal, 1973) - whatever that may mean. There are no effects of atrial receptors on peripheral vessels (Carswell et al., 1970a) or on efferent sympathetic nerves other than those to the sino-atrial node and kidney (Karim et al., 1972). Any reader who looks at all the evidence must come to the conclusion that the stimulation of atrial receptors results only in an increase in heart rate involving only efferent sympathetic nerves and an increase in urine flow.

<u>No Reflex Positive Inotropic Response</u> Because of the known response of the heart to stimulation of efferent sympathetic nerves it was expected that there would be a positive inotropic response as well as

an increase in heart rate when this reflex was evoked. Using dP/dt max to indicate changes in the inotropic state the atrial receptors were again stimulated (Furnival et al., 1971a). We expected to observe a positive inotropic response - in the event there was no positive inotropic response, only an increase in heart rate. The results of 37 experiments in twelve dogs in which the left atrial receptors were stimulated are shown in Fig. 16 in which one response (change in dP/dt max) is plotted against the other (change in heart rate). It can be seen that even with the highest increase in heart rate of 90 beats/min in response to stimulation of left atrial receptors there was an increase of dP/dt max of only 276 mm Hg/sec even less than would have been obtained by simple pacing. The mean change in dP/dt max as a result of stimulating the atrial receptors in the 37 experiments was an increase of 193 mm Hg/sec (mean: range 36-828)- an insignificant amount.

Also shown in Fig. 16, for comparison, is the effect of occluding the carotid arteries in 10 experiments and the effect of an infusion of isoprenaline. It can be seen that with the increase in heart rate resulting from occlusion of the carotid arteries there is a larger increase in dP/dt max; a mean increase of 1263 mm Hg/sec was obtained. The infusion of isoprenaline shows an increase of 3000 mm Hg/sec for an increase of 50 beats/min in the heart rate caused by the isoprenaline in a paced denervated heart (Furnival et al., 1971b).

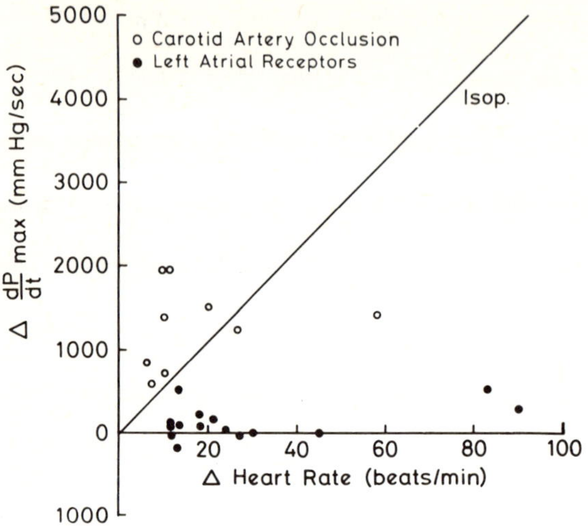

Figure 16.

Change in dP/dt max (positive inotropic effect) plotted against change in heart rate. Filled circles (•) represent responses resulting from the same stimulation of left atrial receptors; open circles (o), responses resulting from carotid occlusion; continuous line, responses resulting from infusions of isoproterenol (Isop.). Note insignificant positive inotropic response to stimulation of left atrial receptors. (From Linden, 1973).

Each of these larger responses indicates that the technique of recording dP/dt max as an index of the inotropic state is valid in this preparation and the increase in dP/dt max in response to stimulation of left atrial receptors is therefore negligible.

So it was concluded that the reflex involved no concomitant inotropic effect - only an increase in heart rate.

Further Evidence in Support of the Atrial Receptor Reflex In another investigation in which an isolated pouch of left atrium containing only the atrial receptors was distended by means of pulsatile changes of pressure Ledsome and Linden (1967) showed that the same reflex response of an increase in the heart rate, could be elicited. Though high pressures were required in the pouch it was later demonstrated (Kidd, Ledsome and Linden, 1966), by recording action potentials in slips of vagal nerves and by the use of the law of La Place, that the tensions in the wall of the pouch, and therefore the stretch of the receptors, would be less even though the pressure in the lumen was higher; the pouch had a radius of curvature about four times less than that of the whole atrium. This investigation served to provide more circumstantial evidence that the atrial receptors were involved in this reflex response. Further experiments showed that the reflex elicited from distension of the pouch had its afferent pathway in the vagal nerves and its efferent pathway only in the sympathetic nerves.

In two other series of experiments in our laboratories (Ledsome and Hainsworth, 1970 ; Carswell et al., 1970a) it was shown that stimulation of the left atrial receptors does not affect either respiration or peripheral resistance. The finding of no effect on the peripheral vessels was supported by the work of Karim et al., (1972) who found that there were no changes in activity in efferent sympathetic nerves in the abdominal sympathetic trunk below the origin of the renal artery when the left atrial receptors were stimulated. However they did find that on stimulating the left atrial receptors they observed that there was an increase in discharge in right ansa subclavia (presumably to the sino-atrial node) but a decrease in discharge in the nerves to the kidney, and no change in any other sympathetic nerves. No function has yet been assigned to the changes in sympathetic nerve activity to the kidney.

In five dogs the preparation was set up again complete with left atrial balloons and then control responses of an increase in heart rate were elicited. The dogs were then made acidotic by inhalation of CO_2 or an infusion of hydrochloric acid and the distensions were repeated. Finally the blood chemistry was brought back to normal again and again the distensions were repeated. It was observed that increasing the acidosis depressed the magnitude of the response obtained from stimulation of left atrial receptors (Harry et al., 1971).

Right Atrial Receptors Using a similar technique and distending the junction of the superior vena cava and the right atrium it has been shown that the same reflex increase in heart rate can be obtained (Kappagoda, Linden and Snow, 1972a and b; Linden, 1973). This reflex was also shown to involve the vagal nerves as the afferent pathway and the sympathetic nerves as the sole efferent pathway of the reflex.

REFLEX DIURESIS

Henry et al., (1956) showed that a large balloon, placed in the left atrium and distended so as to block the mitral orifice and raise the left atrial pressure about 20 cm H_2O, would cause an increase in urine flow. Ledsome and Linden (1968) repeated their experiments and in addition stimulated only the atrial receptors. The results of one experiment is shown in Fig. 17. Two distensions of the large balloon to obstruct the mitral orifice (B) and two distensions of the small balloons to stimulate only the left atrial receptors (A), were completed first. Each distension resulted in an increase in urine flow. Following section of the vagi in the chest at the level of the lung root on the right and at the upper border of the aorta on the left - a procedure which is known to abolish about all the reflex increase in heart rate resulting from stimulation of the left atrial receptors - the response of the increase in urine flow from distension of the large balloon also failed to occur (see Fig. 17, final distension B). The results of nine distensions of the large balloons and nine distensions of the left atrial receptors randomly completed in five dogs showed that the points obtained in both series of experiments appeared to belong to the same

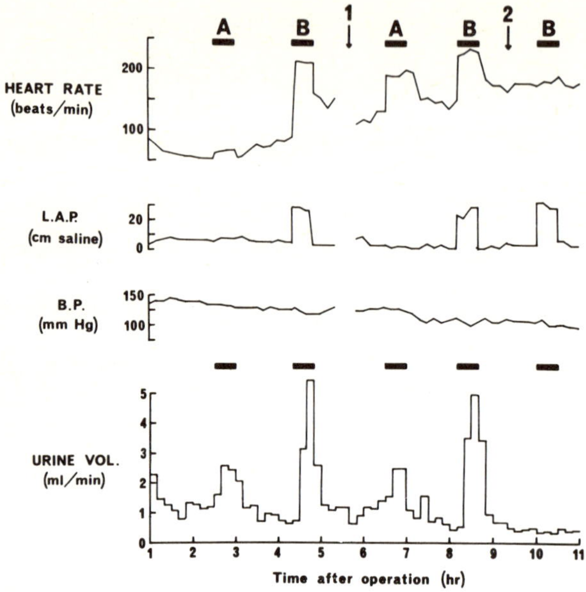

Figure 17.

Changes in urine flow occurring during one experiment in which atrial receptors were stimulated and in which the mitral valve orifice was obstructed. During A, left atrial receptors were stimulated (small balloons at pulmonary vein-atrial junctions). During B, mitral obstruction was caused by large balloon in the manner of Henry et al., (1956). There is a break in the record at "1" where a burst balloon was replaced. At "2" afferent vagal nerves of the heart rate reflex from the left atrial receptors were sectioned. Note that in this instance sectioning the nerves also abolished the diuretic response. L.A.P. = left atrial pressure. (From Ledsome and Linden, 1968).

population. Thus it was concluded that stimulation of the left atrial receptors causes an increase in urine flow, and although the large balloon caused a larger increase in urine output than the smaller ones, there was no reason to believe that the receptors other than atrial receptors were involved: the big balloon was stimulating over a larger area than the smaller ones. Recently Kappagoda, Linden and Snow (1973) reported results of experiments which showed that stretching the right atrium without obstructing venous return or altering right atrial pressure also results in an increase in urine flow in all respects similar to that obtained by stimulating left atrial receptors. Thus we can conclude that both left and right atrial receptors when stimulated cause a diuresis.

From other experiments in our laboratory, with denervated kidneys (Ledsome, Linden and O'Connor, 1961) and perfused kidneys (Carswell et al., 1970) it is possible to conclude that there are two efferent mechanisms involved in this reflex, a blood borne agent and a nervous one, the latter possibly being the sympathetic nerves to the kidney (Karim et al., 1972).

Is The Anti-Diuretic Hormone Involved? Gauer and Henry (1963) postulated that activation of the atrial stretch receptors caused a diuresis by mediating a reflex inhibition of the secretion of anti-diuretic hormone from the post pituitary. This suggestion was made in spite of the report of Ledsome et al., (1961) who showed that the diuresis could be obtained in the presence of large amounts (0.4 m-mu/min) of infused (exogenous) vasopressin, and the suggestion from these authors that the antidiuretic hormone was not involved. However, support for the Gauer and Henry (1963) hypothesis came from Mason and Ledsome (1971), who observed that decreasing a large infusion rate of vasopressin to a smaller but still large infusion rate resulted in a diuresis similar to that observed by distension of balloons in the left atrium. Subsequently Ledsome and Mason (1972) suggested that the diuresis from distension of the left atrium was modified by graded infusions of vasopressin. These experiments could be criticised on the ground that the former (Mason and Ledsome, 1971) bears no relevance to the activities of atrial receptors and the latter (Ledsome and Mason, 1972) merely provides a statistical basis for the inference that the antidiuretic hormone is involved in the response. The above experiments have perpetuated the myth that the concentration of antidiuretic hormone falls in response to distension of the left atrium.

This idea of reflex inhibition of the secretion of antidiuretic hormone from the post pituitary by the atrial receptors has received wide acceptance over the last decade (e.g. Baisset and Montastruc 1957 ; Sjostrand, 1962 ; Woodbury, 1965 ; Shu'ayb, Moran and Zimmerman, 1965 ; Guyton, 1966 ; Nocenti, 1968 ; Zehr, Johnson and Moore, 1969 ; Goetz, Bond, Hemereck and Trank, 1970 ;

Brennan, Malvin, Jochin and Roberts, 1971 ; Ganong, 1971 ; Moore ; 1971 ; Lawrence, Ledsome and Mason, 1973), and became the corner stone of several important reviews on the control of extra-cellular volume (e.g. Share, 1969 ; Gauer, Henry and Behn, 1970 ; Share and Claybaugh, 1972 ; Paintal, 1973). The strength of this belief that ADH was involved in this diuresis is reflected in a recent review by Share and Claybaugh (1972) which states that "the possibility that atrial receptors play no role in the control of vasopressin release is most unlikely in view of the overwhelming evidence that distension of the left atrium can inhibit the release of this hormone." Some of the so-called evidence has been questioned and a discussion of the opinions has been presented (Kappagoda, Linden, Snow and Whitaker, 1974).

Having demonstrated that their bio-assay had sufficient sensitivity to detect changes in concentration of anti-diuretic hormone in the plasma of the unaesthetized dog preparation Kappagoda et al., (1974) examined the effect of distending both the large balloon in the body of the left atrium (in the manner of Henry et al., 1956) and of stimulating only the left atrial receptors on the urine flow and on the level of anti-diuretic activity of the plasma. They obtained a diuresis both by stimulation of the atrial receptors and by distending the large balloon, and they also showed that this diuresis was <u>not</u> accompanied by a reduction in the anti-diuretic activity of the plasma.

Further evidence to support this conclusion was obtained in another series of experiments which have only been reported in a preliminary communication (Kappagoda, Linden, Snow and Whitaker, 1973). Dogs were prepared in the same manner as before, anaesthetized with chloralose, chest opened, a balloon placed in the left atrial appendage and the ureters catheterised. In these dogs the posterior pituitary was ablated. The posterior pituitary was approached through the soft palate. A hole was bored in the sphenoid bone with a dental drill and through it an insulated metal probe was inserted. A diagram is shown in Fig. 18 which illustrates a sagittal view of a dogs head and shows the approach of the probe towards the pituitary fossa. The probe was then advanced 1 cm further than the inner table of the sphenoid bone and a current of 450 mA was passed for 15 sec. The probe was then withdrawn 2 mm a time and at each point the current was passed again. At post mortem the pituitary was observed, both macroscopically and microscopically, to be destroyed. Following the ablation of the pituitary gland and during the whole subsequent experiment no anti-diuretic activity was detectable in the plasma.

Distension of the balloon in the atrium still caused the diuresis in each dog. It was therefore concluded that the diuresis obtainable by stimulation of the atrial receptors is not caused by a reduction in anti-diuretic hormone in the blood.

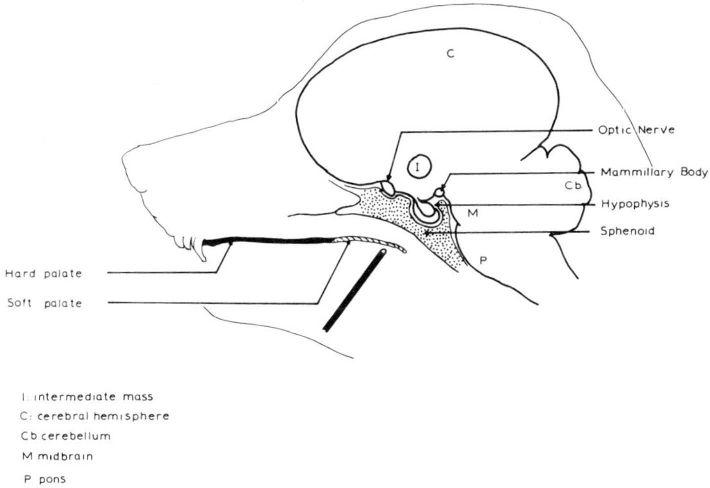

Figure 18.

Diagram of sagittal section of head of dog illustrating point of entry of coagulating probe through the soft palate and sphenoid bone.

It was therefore concluded from these two investigations that, as the agent causing the diuresis was blood borne and was not accompanied by a reduction in anti-diuretic activity, it could only be a diuretic substance.

Speculation relating to Normal Function of Atrial Receptors

This response of an increase in heart rate and an increase in urine flow from left and right atrial receptors has been observed only in dogs and its function in the intact animal and man is unknown. But it is possible to speculate that this reflex is one of the mechanisms which regulates the size of the heart within narrow limits - first by its effect on the heart rate and secondly by its effect on the kidney and the volume of the extra cellular fluid. It is also possible to speculate that these mechanisms may be disarranged in disease. In fact Greenberg et al., (1973) have shown that the atrial receptors discharge less in dogs with chronic heart failure than in normal dogs even though the atrial pressures are higher in the dogs with heart failure. This effect of less atrial receptor discharge may be causative in relation to the known increase in extracellular liquid in heart failure - but it may be the result of heart failure. These speculations and argument leading to them have been discussed (Linden, 1973).

Acknowledgements

I would like to thank the members of the Cardiovascular Unit, University of Leeds for much helpful discussion and comment and particularly my colleague Dr. C.T. Kappagoda who has shared equally in so much of the research and discussion. Most of the work was completed with financial help from the British Heart Foundation, the Medical Research Council, and Wellcome Trust.

REFERENCES

Angell James, J.E. and Daly, M. de B. (1970). Comparison of the reflex vasomotor responses to separate and combined stimulation of the carotid sinus and aortic arch baroreceptors by pulsatile and non-pulsatile pressures in the dog. J. Physiol. 209, 257-293.

Bainbridge, F.A. (1915). The influence of venous filling upon the rate of the heart. J. Physiol. 50, 65-84.

Baisset, A. and Montastruc, P. (1957). Polyurie par distension auriculaire chez le chien; role de l'hormone antidiuretique. J. Physiol. Paris 49, 33-36.

Baker, D., Ellis, R.M., Franklin, D.L. and Rushmer, R.F. (1959). Some engineering aspects of modern cardiac research. Proc. Inst. Radio Engrs. N.Y. 47, 1917-1924.

Berkley, H.J. (1895). The intrinsic nerve supply of the cardiac ventricles in certain vertibrates. Johns Hopkins Hosp. Reports 4, 248-274.

Bezold, A. von (1863). Untersuchungen uber die Innervation des Herzens. Vol. 2, 191, Engelmann, Leipzig.

Braunwald, E. (1965). The control of ventricular function in man. Brit. Heart J. 27, 1-16.

Brennan, L.A., Malvin, R.L., Jochim, K.E. and Roberts, D.E. (1971). Influence of right and left atrial receptors on plasma concentrations of ADH and renin. Amer. J. Physiol. 221, 273-278.

Burkhart, S.M. and Ledsome, J.R. (1974). The response to distension of the pulmonary vein-left atrial junctions in dogs with spinal section. J. Physiol. 237, 685-700.

Carswell, F., Hainsworth, R. and Ledsome, J.R. (1970a). The effects of distension of the pulmonary vein-atrial junctions upon peripheral resistance. J. Physiol. 207, 1-14.

Carswell, F., Hainsworth, R. and Ledsome, J.R. (1970b). The effects of left atrial distension upon urine flow from the isolated perfused kidney. Quart. J. Exp. Physiol. 55, 173-182.

Daly, I de B. and Daly, M. de B. (1959). The effects of stimulation of the carotid sinus baroreceptors on the pulmonary vascular bed in the dog. J. Physiol. 148, 220-226.

Daly, M. de B., Hazzledine, J.L. and Howe, A. (1965). Reflex respiratory and peripheral vascular responses to stimulation of the isolated perfused aortic arch chemoreceptors of dogs. J. Physiol. 177, 300-322.

De Geest, H., Levy, M.N. and Zieske, H. Jr. (1965). Reflex effects of cephalic hypoxia, hypercapnia and ischemia upon ventricular contractility. Circ. Res. 17, 349-358.

Donald, D.E. and Edis, A.J. (1971). Comparison of aortic and carotid baroreflexes in the dog. J. Physiol. 215, 521-538.

Downing, S.E. and Gardner, T.H. (1968). Cephalic and carotid reflex influences on cardiac function. Amer. J. Physiol. 215, 1192-1199.

Downing, S.E., Mitchell, J.H. and Wallace, A.G. (1963). Cardiovascular responses to ischaemia, hypoxia and hypercapnia of the central nervous system. Amer. J. Physiol. 204, 881-887.

Edis, A.J., Donald, D.E. and Shepherd, J.T. (1970). Cardio-vascular reflexes from stretch of pulmonary vein-atrial junctions in the dog. Circ. Res. 27, 1091-1100.

Edis, A.J. and Shepherd, J.T. (1969). Circulatory reflexes from stretch of pulmonary vein-atrial junctions. Physiologist, 12, No. 3. 213.

Floyd, K., Linden, R.J. and Saunders, D.A. (1972). Presumed receptors in the left atrial appendage of the dog. J. Physiol. 227, 27-28P.

Furnival, C.M., Linden, R.J. and Snow, H.M. (1970). Inotropic changes in the left ventricle: the effect of changes in heart rate, aortic pressure and end-diastolic pressure. J. Physiol. 211, 359-387.

Furnival, C.M., Linden, R.J. and Snow, H.M. (1971a). Reflex effects on the heart of stimulating left atrial receptors. J. Physiol. 218, 447-463.

Furnival, C.M., Linden, R.J. and Snow, H.M. (1971b). The inotropic and chronotropic effects of catecholamines on the dog heart. J. Physiol. 214, 15-28.

Furnival, C.M., Linden, R.J. and Snow, H.M. (1973a). The inotropic effect on the heart of stimulating the vagus in the dog, duck and toad. J. Physiol. 230, 155-170.

Furnival, C.M., Linden, R.J. and Snow, H.M. (1973b). Chronotropic and inotropic effects on the dog heart of stimulating the efferent cardiac sympathetic nerves. J. Physiol. 230, 137-153.

Ganong, W.F. (1971). Review of Medical Physiology, 5th edn., p.164. Los Altos: Lange Medical Publications.

Gaskell, W.H. (1900). The contraction of cardiac muscle. In "Schafer's Textbook of Physiology." Vol. 2, p. 169. Pentland, Edinburgh.

Gauer, O.H. and Henry, J.P. (1963). Circulatory basis of fluid volume control. Physiol. Rev. 43, 423-481.

Gauer, O.H., Henry, J.P. and Behn, C. (1970). The regulation of extracellular fluid volume. A. Rev. Physiol. 32, 547-595.

Greenberg, T.T., Richmond, W.H., Stocking, R.A., Gupta, P.D., Meehan, J.P. and Henry, J.P. (1973). Impaired atrial receptor responses in dogs with heart failure due to tricuspid insufficiency and aortic stenosis. Circ. Res. 32, 424-433.

Goetz, K.L., Bond, G.C., Hemreck, A.S. and Trank, J.W. (1970). Plasma ADH levels following a decrease in mean atrial transmural pressure in dogs. Amer. J. Physiol. 219, 1424-1428.

Guyton, A.C. (1966). Textbook of Medical Physiology, 3rd edn., p. 504, Philadelphia and London: W.B. Saunders Co.

Hainsworth, R., Ledsome, J.R. and Carswell, F. (1970). Reflex responses from aortic barareceptors. Amer. J. Physiol. 218, 423-429.

Hainsworth, R. and Karim, F. (1972). Inotropic responses of the left ventricle to changes in aortic arch pressure in anaesthetized dogs. J. Physiol. 223, 213-228.

Hainsworth, R. and Karim, F. (1973). Left ventricular inotropic and peripheral vasomotor responses from independent changes in pressure in the carotid sinuses and cerebral arteries in anaesthetized dogs. J. Physiol. 228, 139-155.

Harry, J.D., Kappagoda, C.T., Linden, R.J. and Snow, H.M. (1971). Depression of the reflex tachycardia from the left atrial receptors by acidaemia. J. Physiol. 218, 465-475.

Henry, J.P., Gauer, O.H. and Reeves, J.L. (1956). Evidence of the atrial location of receptors influencing urine flow. Circ. Res. 4, 85-90.

Heymans, C. and Neil, E. (1958). Reflexogenic Areas of the Cardiovascular System, London, Churchill.

Hunt, R. (1899). Direct and reflex acceleration of the mammalian heart with some observations on the relations of the inhibitory and accelerator nerves. Amer. J. Physiol. 2, 395-470.

Johnston, B.D. (1968). Nerve endings in the human endocardium. Amer. J. Anat. 122, 621-630.

Kappagoda, C.T., Linden, R.J. and Snow, H.M. (1972a). A reflex increase in heart rate from distension of the junction between the superior vena cava and the right atrium. J. Physiol. 220, 177-197.

Kappagoda, C.T., Linden, R.J. and Snow, H.M. (1972b). The effect of stretching the superior vena caval-right atrial junction on right atrial receptors in the dog. J. Physiol. 227, 875-887.

Kappagoda, C.T., Linden, R.J. and Snow, H.M. (1973). Effect of stimulating right atrial receptors on urine flow in the dog. J. Physiol. 235, 493-502.

Kappagoda, C.T., Linden, R.J. and Snow, H.M. and Whitaker, E.M. (1973). Left atrial receptors and diuresis in the dog. J. Physiol. 237, 48–49P.

Kappagoda, C.T., Linden, R.J., Snow, H.M. and Whitaker, E.M. (1974). Left atrial receptors and the antidiuretic hormone. J. Physiol. 237, 663–683.

Karim, F., Kidd, C., Malpus, C.M. and Penna, P.E. (1972). The effects of stimulation of the left atrial receptors on sympathetic efferent nerve fibres. J. Physiol. 227, 243–260.

Kidd, C., Ledsome, J.R. and Linden, R.J. (1966). Left atrial receptors and the heart rate. J. Physiol. 185, 78P.

Lawrence, M., Ledsome, J.R. and Mason, J.M. (1973). The time course of the diuretic response to left atrial distension. Q. Jl. exp. Physiol. 58, 219–227.

Ledsome, J.R. and Hainsworth, R. (1970). The effects upon respiration of distension of the pulmonary vein-atrial junctions. Resp. Physiol. 9, 86-94.

Ledsome, J.R., Linden, R.J. and O'Connor, W.J. (1961). The mechanisms by which distension of the left atrium produces diuresis in anaesthetized dogs. J. Physiol. 159, 87-100.

Ledsome, J.R. and Linden, R.J. (1964a). A reflex increase in heart rate from distension of the pulmonary vein-atrial junctions. J. Physiol. 170, 456-473.

Ledsome, J.R. and Linden, R.J. (1964b). The effect of bretylium tosylate on some cardiovascular reflexes. J. Physiol. 170, 442-455.

Ledsome, J.R. and Linden, R.J. (1967). The effect of distending a pouch of the left atrium on the heart rate. J. Physiol. 193, 121-129.

Ledsome, J.R. and Linden, R.J. (1968). The role of the left atrial receptors in the diuretic response to left atrial distension. J. Physiol. 198, 487-503.

Ledsome, J.R. and Mason, J.M. (1972). The effects of vasopressin on the diuretic response to left atrial distension. J. Physiol. 221, 427-440.

Levy, M.N., Ng, M.L. and Zieske, H. (1966). Cardiac and respiratory effects of aortic arch baroreceptor stimulation. Circ. Res. 19, 930-939.

Linden, R.J. (1963). The control of the output of the heart. In "Recent Advances in Physiology." Edited by R. Creese. Churchill, London.

Linden, R.J. (1968). The heart - ventricular function. Anaesthesia 23, 566-584.

Linden, R.J. (1972). Function of nerves of the heart. Cardiovasc. Res. 6, 605-626.

Linden, R.J. (1973). Function of cardiac receptors. Circulation 48, 463-480.

Mason, J.M. and Ledsome, J.R. (1971). The effect of changes in the rate of infusion of vasopressin in the anaesthetized dog. Can. J. Physiol. Pharmacol. 49, 933-940.

Miller, M.R. and Kasahara, M. (1964). Studies of nerve endings in the heart. Amer. J. Anat. 115, 217-234.

Mizeres, N.J. (1955). The anatomy of the autonomic system in the dog. Amer. J. Anat. 96, 285-302.

Mizeres, N.J. (1958). The origin and course of cardio accelerator fibres in the dog. Anat. Rec. 132, 261-278.

Moore, W.M. (1971). The hypophysis. In "Physiology" (E.E. Selkurt, ed), 3rd edn., p.725. Boston, Little, Brown and Co.

Nocenti, M.R. (1968). Pituitary gland. In "Medical Physiology" (V.B. Mountcastle, ed), 12th edn., vol. 1, p.894. Saint Louis, The C.V. Mosby Co.

Nonidez, J.R. (1939). Studies on the innervation of the heart. Distribution of cardiac nerves with special reference to identification of sympathetic and parasympathetic post-ganglionics. Amer. J. Anat. 65, 361-413.

Paintal, A.S. (1973). Vagal sensory receptors and their reflex effects. Physiol. Rev. 53, 159-227.

Randall, W.C. and Rohse, W.G. (1956). The agumentor action of the sympathetic cardiac nerves. Circ. Res. 22, 315-323.

Randall, W.C., Wechsler, J.S., Pace, J.B. and Szentivanyi, M. (1968). Alterations in myocardial contractility during stimulation of the cardiac nerves. Amer. J. Physiol. 214, 1205-1212.

Rushmer, R.F. and West, T.C. (1956). Cardiac responses to sympathetic stimulation. Circ. Res. 4, 302-307.

Sagawa, K., Ross, J.M. and Guyton, A.G. (1961). Quantitation of cerebral ischemia pressor response in dogs.
Amer. J. Physiol. 200, 1164-1168.

Sarnoff, S.J., Brockman, S.K., Gilmore, J.P., Linden, R.J. and Mitchell, J.H. (1960). Regulation of ventricular contraction. Influence of cardiac sympathetic and vagal nerve stimulation on atrial and ventricular dynamics. Circ. Res. 8, 1108-1122.

Share, L. (1969). Extracellular fluid volume and vasopressin secretion. In "Frontiers in Neuroendocrinology" (W.F. Ganong and L. Martini, eds), New York, Oxford Univ. Press.

Share, L. and Claybaugh, J.R. (1972). Regulation of body fluids. A. Rev. Physiol. 34, 235-260.

Sjostrand, T. (1962). Blood Volume. In "Circulation" (W.F. Hamilton and P. Dow, eds) 1st edn., vol. 1, pp. 51-62. Washington, American Physiological Society.

Shu'ayb, W.A., Moran, W.H. and Zimmerman, B. (1965). Studies of the mechanism of antidiuretic hormone secretion and post-commissurotomy dilutional syndrome. Ann. Surg. 162, 690-701.

Woodbury, D.M. (1965). Physiology of body fluids. In "Physiology and Biophysics" (T.C. Ruch and H.D. Patton, eds), 19th edn., p.895. Philadelphia and London, W.B. Saunders, Co.

Zehr, J.E., Johnson, J.A. and Moore, W.W. (1969). Left atrial pressure, plasma osmolality and ADH levels in the unanaesthetized ewe. Amer. J. Physiol. 217, 1672-1680.

Actions of Catecholamines on Ionic Currents in Cardiac Muscle

D. NOBLE

University Department of Physiology, Oxford, U.K.

IONIC MECHANISM OF ACTION POTENTIAL

Before discussing the actions of catecholamines, it is necessary to describe the ionic conductance changes that underly the electrical events. I shall do this fairly briefly here since a detailed account will be found elsewhere (Noble, 1975).

It has been known for some years that the initial rapid depolarization is attributable to a large and transient increase in sodium conductance similar to that observed in nerve cells (see Weidmann, 1955 ; Beeler and Reuter, 1970a ; Dudel and Rudel, 1970). It is also probable that this conductance persists at a very low level during the plateau of the action potential since such a residual conductance is predicted by the Hodgkin-Huxley equations (see Noble, 1966). Early models of the cardiac action potential (e.g. Noble, 1962) attributed the maintenance of the plateau to this residual sodium conductance but it is now clear that this is only partly true. The plateau is also maintained by the activation of a smaller inward conductance attributable to the flow of calcium ions. (Beeler and Reuter, 1970b ; New and Trautwein, 1972). This current flow not only helps to maintain the plateau, it is also an important link in the coupling process between excitation and contraction. (Beeler and Reuter, 1970c ; Vassort, 1974).

The outward (repolarizing) currents in cardiac membranes differ very markedly indeed from those in nerve membranes. This is not surprising in view of the very large differences between the repolarization process in the two tissues.

The first effect of depolarization is to <u>reduce</u> the potassium conductance of the membrane (Hall, Hutter and Noble, 1963 ; Deck and Trautwein, 1964 ; Hutter and Noble, 1960 ; Carmeliet, 1961). This fall is attributable to the presence of inward rectification and the consequences of this kind of rectification are important in interpreting the effects of potassium concentration changes on electrical activity in the heart (see Noble, 1965). The fact that g_k is low during the plateau also helps to explain the high membrane resistance that occurs at this time (Weidmann, 1951 ; Noble and Tsien, 1972) and it ensures that relatively small inward currents are sufficient to maintain the plateau which is obviously advantageous from an energetic point of view.

The second effect of depolarization is to activate time-dependent potassium currents. These currents are involved partly in repolarization (though much of this is also attributable to a steady decrease in calcium current flow). The relative contributions of potassium activation and calcium inactivation to controlling the duration of the cardiac action potential is variable and may differ quite substantially in different parts of the heart.

The other role of the time-dependent potassium currents is that they control the rate of pacemaker activity (Noble and Tsien, 1968 ; Brown, Clark and Noble, 1972). This will be particularly important in the present context since the actions of catecholamines that I shall discuss are the chronotropic actions.

Fig. 1 summarizes the current changes underlying the action potential and the pacemaker depolarization.

The ionic mechanisms underlying the inhibitory action of acetylcholine on cardiac muscle have been known for some time (see review by Hutter, 1957). The action is to increase the potassium permeability of the membrane in a highly specific way and so produce an inhibitory hyper-polarization similar to that observed at some central nervous inhibitory

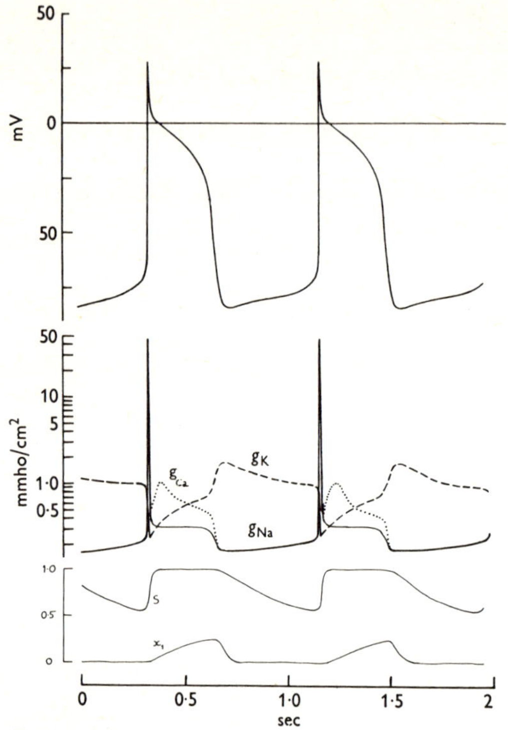

Figure 1

synapses. By contrast, the ionic mechanism of the excitatory actions of adrenaline and other catecholamines have remained mysterious until recently.

The reason for this situation is that the actions of adrenaline are unusual from a synaptic point of view since they have been found to involve changes in the behaviour of the voltage and time-dependent conductances underlying the non-linear properties of the membrane. Their elucidation has therefore awaited the application of voltage clamp techniques to cardiac cells. Moreover, the mechanisms by which acceleration occurs are very different in different parts of the heart. The two main preparations that have been studied and which show pacemaker activity are mamallian Purkinje fibres and frog atrial trabeculae. The latter show pacemaker activity in response to small depolarizing currents and this response strongly resembles spontaneous pacemaker activity in sinus tissue. Both preparations show similar potential changes on exposure to adrenaline, i.e. an acceleration of pacemaker depolarization and an increase in the maximum diastolic potential. The acceleration in frog atrium is however not always so pronounced as it is in the Purkinje fibre and the reasons for this lie in the fact that the ionic current changes responsible are quite different.

PACEMAKER MECHANISM IN PURKINJE FIBRES

Noble and Tsien (1968) analysed the kinetics of a potassium current, i_{K_2}, whose decay following each action potential is responsible for the pacemaker depolarization in Purkinje fibres (Deck and Trautwein, 1964 ; Vassalle, 1966). This current is activated by a gating mechanism, s, whose threshold lies at -90 mV and which becomes fully-activated in the steady state at -60 mV. This is also the range of potentials over which the pacemaker depolarization occurs, which means that the activation of the current i_{K_2} is strongly voltage dependent in this range.

During each action potential s becomes fully-activated since the time constant of activation during strong depolarizations is very short compared to the duration of the action potential (McAllister and Noble, 1966). The pacemaker depolarization therefore starts at a time when all the i_{K_2} channels are open. The time constant of decay of s at potentials in the pacemaker range is 1 or 2 seconds. As this decay occurs, the magnitude of the potassium current decreases so allowing an inward background current to depolarize the membrane. During a single pacemaker potential the number of i_{K_2} channels activated decays by about 50%.

One of the factors that limits the speed at which the decay occurs, and hence the frequency of beating, is the position of the steady state activation curve. At the beginning of the depolarization, when the membrane potential lies near the threshold for activation of i_{K_2}, the degree of activation falls fairly rapidly as s moves from full activation towards zero activation. As the depolarization occurs, however, the steady state degree of activation increases and so the value towards which s moves increases. The rate of decay of s therefore decreases. Indeed, as shown in Figure 2, the rate of decay becomes zero when $s = s_\infty$. Beyond this point the channels begin to open up again and it is only the highly non-linear behaviour of the channels themselves (which show inward-rectification and so carry much less current as the membrane becomes depolarized), and the activation

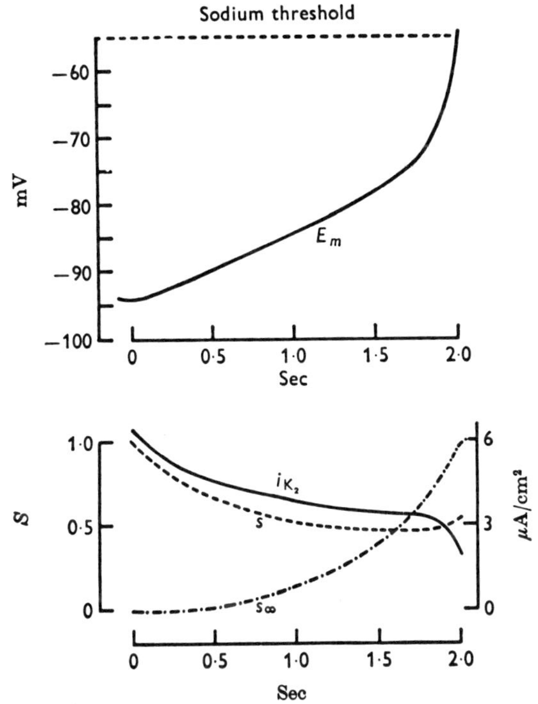

Figure 2

of inward sodium current as the threshold is approached that allows the depolarization to continue beyond this point (see McAllister, Noble and Tsien, 1974).

MECHANISM OF ACCELERATION IN PURKINJE FIBRES

The fact that the position of the activation curve for s limits the rate of decay of i_{K_2} suggests a way in which acceleration could be achieved. This is to shift the activation curve in a depolarizing direction, i.e. raise its threshold, so that the steady state value at

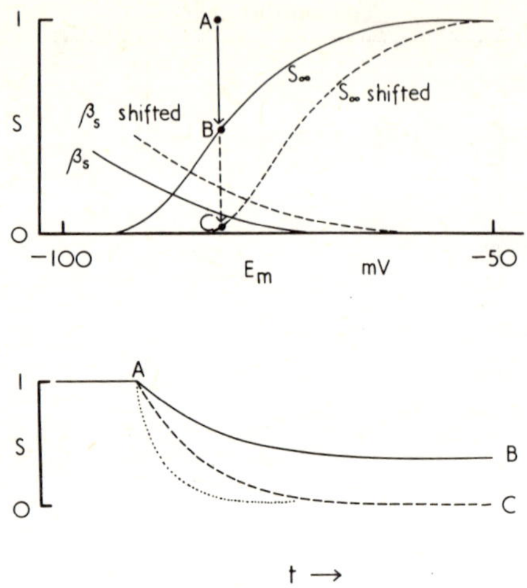

Figure 3

potentials in the pacemaker range is reduced. As shown in Fig. 3 this would be a powerful way of producing acceleration. If the time constant of decay were unaltered, the decay would be more rapid from A to C than from A to B since a larger absolute change is involved; the degree of activation decays towards a lower value (interrupted curve). In fact, the mechanism of acceleration would be even more powerful since the time constant of decay becomes much shorter as the membrane is hyperpolarized. If the time constant curve is also shifted (as is likely since, in a Hodgkin-Huxley mechanism) the time constant and activation curves are closely related) the increase in rate of decay will be even greater (dotted line).

An experiment to test the possibility that a shift in the s

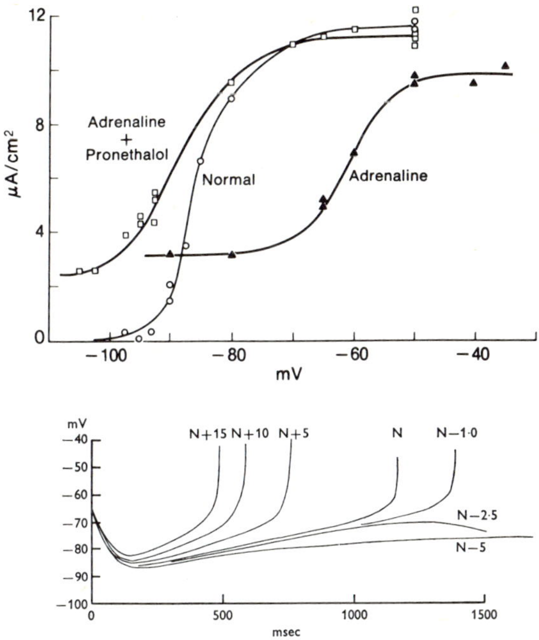

Figure 4

activation curve occurs in the presence of adrenaline was performed by Hauswirth, Noble and Tsien and is illustrated in Fig. 4. Here it can be seen that the action of adrenaline does indeed shift the activation curve in a depolarizing direction and that this action may be reversed by the β-blocker pronethalol. The lower part of this figure shows the results of some computer calculations done to test whether the observed shifts are adequate to account for the acceleration produced. Curve N shows the pacemaker depolarization computed from a model of the ionic currents analysed by voltage clamp techniques (see Hauswirth, McAllister, Noble and Tsien, 1969 ; McAllister, Noble and Tsien, 1974). The other curves show the pacemaker potentials computed after introducing various degrees of shift (in mV). It is clear that even quite small shifts in a depolarizing direction produce a marked degree of acceleration.

*PACEMAKER MECHANISM IN ATRIAL FIBRES

It is difficult to perform voltage clamp experiments on the natural pacemaker, the sino-atrial node, and as yet, only one report has appeared (Irisawa, 1972). This suggests that the mechanism involved is similar to that in Purkinje fibres. In this section we shall explain the reasons against this view, although we agree with Irisawa that a potassium conductance decay is involved.

Quiescent frog atrial trabeculae (on which it is much easier to perform voltage clamp experiments - Rougier, Vassort and Stämpfli, 1968 ; Brown and Noble, 1969) may often be made to generate pacemaker activity very similar to that in the SA node by applying small steady depolarizing currents. This is illustrated in Fig. 5. When the current level indicated by the interrupted line is maintained the membrane fires repetitively. The major difference between the pacemaker activity in sinus and atrial tissue and that in

* I am grateful to Dr. Hilary Brown and Dr. Susan Noble for the material described in this section, which is taken from Brown et al., 1974.

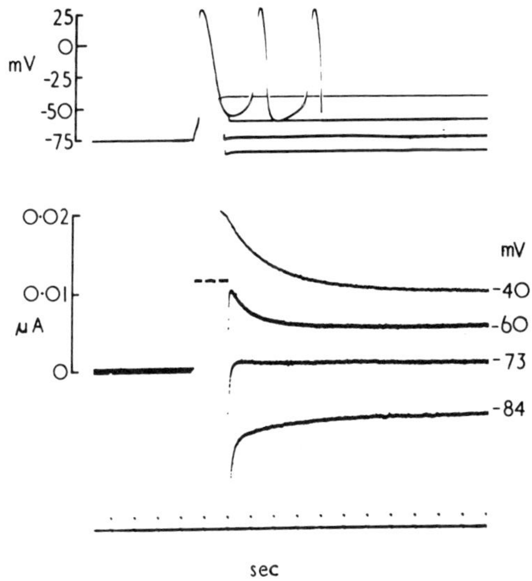

Figure 5

Purkinje fibres lies in the fact that the potential range over which pacemaker activity occurs is quite different. As we have already noted, the pacemaker depolarization in Purkinje fibres runs from about −90 mV to about −60 mV (Fig. 1), whereas in atrial fibres the pacemaker range is usually positive to −60 mV (Fig. 5). Since s is fully activated in the steady state at potentials positive to −60 mV, one would not expect variations in a current controlled by s to be involved. Moreover, little or no delayed potassium current is activated in the s range on atrial fibres (Brown, Clark and Noble, 1974a, b). It is quite possible, therefore, that the s mechanism does not exist in these fibres.

Nevertheless, a potassium conductance of some kind is involved in pacemaker activity. This is illustrated by the experiment by Brown, Clark and Noble shown in Fig. 5. At the termination of the first action potential the voltage clamp was applied at various potentials. At potentials positive to -73 mV the result is a decaying outward current. At potentials negative to this value, a decaying inward current is observed. This suggests that a potassium current is involved but that its reversal potential is significantly positive to E_K, which is probably near -90 mV (Haas, Glitsch and Kern, 1966). This contrasts with the properties of i_{K_2} in the Purkinje fibre which reverses very near to E_K (Noble and Tsien, 1968 ; Peper and Trautwein, 1969). The atrial pacemaker K^+ mechanism is therefore less highly selective than that in Purkinje fibres.

A less selective K current mechanism is in fact displayed by Purkinje fibres but the activation range lies substantially positive to that for i_{K_2} and it is not normally involved in pacemaker activity. This mechanism was called i_x by Noble and Tsien (1969) to indicate that some ions other than potassium must also be transported to a small extent. The activation threshold for i_x lies at about -40 mV, which is 50 mV more positive than that for i_{K_2}.

The actovation curve for the atrial potassium current also lies at similar potentials (see Fig. 6). These observations suggest that it is

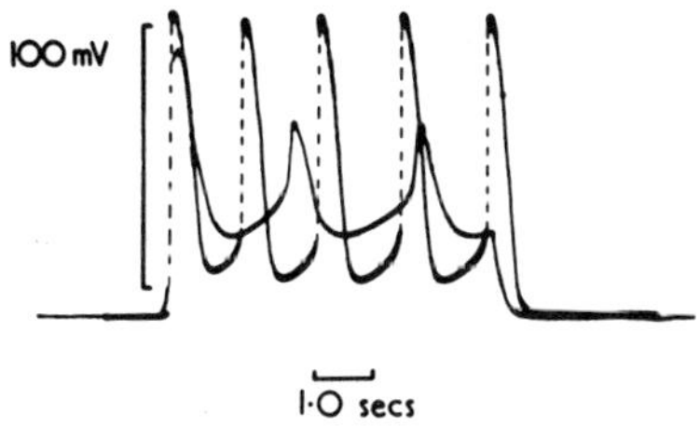

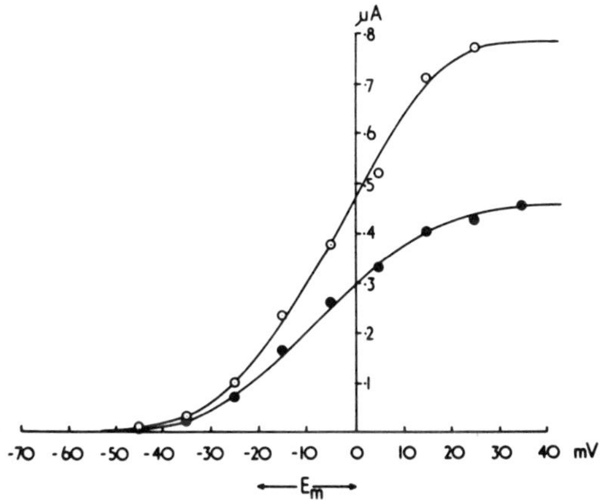

Figure 6

comparable to i_x in Purkinje fibres and not to i_{K_2}. We shall present further evidence for this view when the actions of adrenaline have been discussed.

MECHANISM OF ACCELERATION IN ATRIAL FIBRES

Fig. 6 (top) shows induced atrial pacemaker potentials before and after the addition of adrenaline to the Ringer's solution. It can be seen that when adrenaline is present the action potential height is increased, the repolarization is more rapid, the potential then reaches a more negative level and the pacemaker depolarization which follows is more rapid. It is clear from Fig. 4 that not all of these changes could be reproduced by a simple depolarizing shift of the potassium activation curve.

In fact, none of the changes seen in Fig. 6 (top) are attributable to a potassium threshold shift since the threshold for i_x is unaltered by adrenaline (Fig. 5 bottom). Instead, the <u>magnitude</u> of the current is increased. This contrasts very strongly with the action on the pacemaker K current, i_{K_2}, in Purkinje fibres, although it partly resembles the action of adrenaline on the current i_x in Purkinje fibres. Here also an increase in magnitude is seen (Tsien, Giles and Greengard, 1972 ; McNaughton, 1974).

These results further strengthen the identification of the atrial pacemaker current with i_x. They also go some way towards explaining the actions of adrenaline on atrial fibres. The increased rate of repolarization and the increased maximum negative potential are both explained by a larger K current activated during the action potential.

However, by themselves, these effects would have a decelerating effect since a larger K current will take longer to decay and should therefore lead to a prolonged interval between action potentials. There must therefore be an effect of adrenaline on another current component. The obvious choice is the calcium current, which

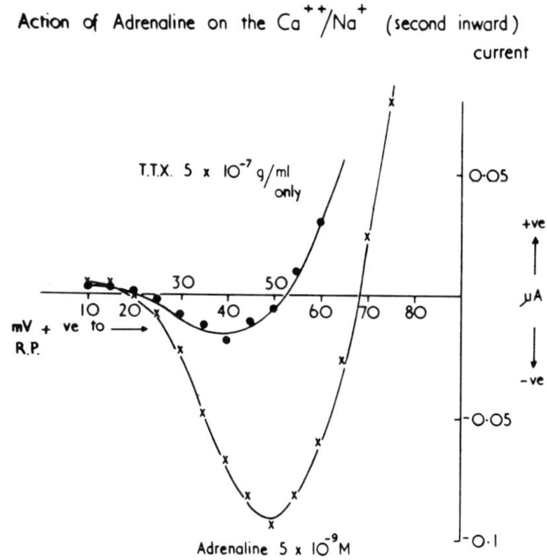

Figure 7

is known to be increased by adrenaline (Rougier, Vassort, Garnier, Gargouil and Coraboeuf, 1969). If a large enough increase in inward calcium current were to occur, the pacemaker depolarization would be accelerated as it approaches the calcium threshold. As shown in Fig. 7, the increase in calcium current produced by adrenaline can sometimes be extremely large and is large enough to allow pacemaker activity and action potentials to occur when the sodium current is blocked by tetrodotoxin. It is certain therefore that the calcium current can be involved in pacemaker activity (see also Lenfant, Mironneau and Aka, 1972).

In view of the fact that normal repetitive activity in the SA node occurs over a potential range similar to that into which atrial preparations must be depolarized to produce pacemaker activity it seems likely that here also the pacemaker mechanism may be attributable to decay of i_x and that the mechanisms of actions of adrenaline resemble those induced atrial pacemakers. In this connection it is interesting to note that Purkinje fibres may also show pacemaker activity at less negative potentials than normal under many circumstances (e.g. anoxia, low $[K]_o$ and high doses of cardiac glycosides). In these cases the pacemaker activity resembles that of induced atrial activity and the potassium current involved is i_x rather than i_{K_2} (Hauswirth, Noble and Tsien, 1969).

REFERENCES

Beeler, G.W. and Reuter, H. (1970a). Voltage clamp experiments on ventricular myocardial fibres. J. Physiol. 207, 165-190

Beeler, G.W. and Reuter, H. (1970b). Membrane calcium current in ventricular myocardial fibres. J. Physiol. 207, 191-209

Beeler, G.W. and Reuter, H. (1970c). The relation between membrane potential, membrane currents and activation of contraction in ventricular myocardial fibres. J. Physiol. 207, 211-229

Brown, H.F., Clark, A. and Noble, S.J. (1972). The pacemaker current in frog atrium. Nature New Biology 235, 30-31

Brown, H.F., Clark, A. and Noble, S.J. (1974a). Identification of the pacemaker current in frog atrium (submitted to J. Physiol.)

Brown, H.F., Clark, A. and Noble, S.J. (1974b). Voltage clamp analysis of an atrial pacemaker current (submitted to J. Physiol.)

Brown, H.F., McNaughton, P.A., Noble, D. and Noble, S.J. (1974). Adrenergic control of cardiac pacemaker currents. Phil.Trans. Roy. Soc. (in press).

Brown, H.F. and Noble, S.J. (1969a). Membrane currents underlying delayed rectification and pacemaker activity in frog atrial muscle. J. Physiol. 204, 717-736.

Brown, H.F. and Noble, S.J. (1969b). A quantitative analysis of the slow component of delayed rectification in frog atrium. J. Physiol. 204, 737-747.

Brown, R.H. and Noble, D. (1974). The influence of protons and calcium ions on membrane currents in cardiac Purkinje fibres. (Submitted to J. Physiol.).

Carmeliet, E. (1961). Chloride ions and the membrane potential of Purkinje fibres. J. Physiol. 156, 375-388.

Deck, K.A. and Trautwein, W. (1964). Ionic currents in cardiac excitation. Pflügers Arch. 280, 65-80.

Dudel, J. and Rudel, R. (1970). Voltage and time dependence of sodium current in cooled sheep Purkinje fibres. Pflügers Arch. 315, 136-158.

Haas, H.G., Glitsch, H.G. and Kern, R. (1966). Kalium-Fluxe und Membranpotential am Froschvorhof in Abhangigheit von der Kalium-Aussen-konzentration. Pflügers Arch. 288, 43-64.

Hall, A.E., Hutter, O.F. and Noble, D. (1963). Current-voltage relations of Purkinje fibres in sodium-deficient solutions. J. Physiol. 166, 225-240.

Hauswirth, O., McAllister, R.E., Noble, D. and Tsien, R.W. (1969). Reconstruction of the actions of adrenaline and calcium ions on cardiac pacemaker potentials. J. Physiol, 126-128P.

Hauswirth, O., Noble, D. and Tsien, R.W. (1968). Adrenaline: mechanism of action on the pacemaker potential in cardiac Purkinje fibres. Science, 162, 916-917.

Hauswirth, O., Noble, D. and Tsien, R.W. (1969). The mechanism of oscillatory activity at low membrane potentials in cardiac Purkinje fibres. J. Physiol. 200, 255-265

Hutter, O.F. (1957). Mode of action of autonomic transmitters on the Heart. Brit. Med. Bull. 13, 176-180.

Hutter, O.F. and Noble, D. (1960). Rectifying properties of cardiac muscle Nature 188, 495.

Irisawa, H. (1972). Electrical activity of rabbit sino-atrial node. In: Symposium on the electrical field of the heart. (Ed. P. Rijlant). Brussels: Presses Academiques Europeennes.

Lenfant, J., Mironneau, J. and Aka, J.K. (1972). Activité répétitive de la fibre sino-auriculaire de grenouille: Analyse des courants membranaires responsables de l'automatisme cardiaque. J. Physiol. (Paris) 64, 5-18.

McAllister, R.E. and Noble, D. (1966). The time and voltage dependence of the slow outward current in cardiac Purkinje fibres. J. Physiol. 186, 632-662.

McAllister, R.E., Noble, D. and Tsien, R.W. (1974). Reconstruction of the electrical activity of cardiac Purkinje fibres. (submitted to J. Physiol.)

McNaughton, P.A. (1974). The relation between intracellular calcium ion concentration and the chronotropic action of adrenaline in cardiac Purkinje fibres (submitted to J. Physiol.)

New, W. and Trautwein, W. (1972a). Inward membrane currents in mammalian myocardium. Pflügers Arch. 334, 1-23.

New, W. and Trautwein, W. (1972b). The ionic nature of slow inward current and its relation to contraction. Pflügers Arch. 334, 24-38.

Noble, D. (1962a). A modification of the Hodgkin-Huxley equations applicable to Purkinje Fibre action and pacemaker potentials. J. Physiol. 160, 317-352.

Noble, D. (1962b). Computed action potentials and their experimental basis. Proc. Int. Union Physiol. Sci. 1, 177-182

Noble, D. (1962c). The voltage dependence of the cardiac membrane conductance. Biophys J. 2, 381-393.

Noble, E. (1965). Electrical properties of cardiac muscle attributable to inward-going (anomalous) rectification. J. cell. comp. Physiol. 66 (Suppl 2.) 127-136.

Noble, D. (1966). Applications of the Hodgkin-Huxley equations to excitable tissues. Physiol. Rev. 46, 1-50.

Noble, D. (1974). Cardiac action potentials and pacemaker activity. Recent advances in Physiology. pp. 1 (Ed. R.J. Linden). London : Churchill.

Noble, D. (1975). The Initiation of the Heartbeat, Oxford. The Clarendon Press.

Noble, D. and Tsien, R.W. (1968). The kinetics and rectifier properties of the slow potassium current in cardiac Purkinje fibres. J. Physiol. 195, 185-214.

Noble, D. and Tsien, R.W. (1969a). Outward membrane currents activated in the plateau range of potentials in cardiac Purkinje Fibres. J. Physiol. 200, 205-231.

Noble, D. and Tsien, R.W. (1969b). Reconstruction of the repolarization process in cardiac Purkinje fibres based on voltage clamp measurements of the membrane current. J. Physiol. 200, 233-254.

Noble, E. and Tsien, R.W. (1972). The repolarization process of heart cells. In: Electrical phenomena in the heart, pp. 133-161. (Ed. De Mello). New York: Academic Press.

Peper, K. and Trautwein, W. (1969). A note on the pacemaker current in Purkinje fibres. Pflügers Arch. 309, 356-361.

Rougier, O., Vassort, G. and Stampfli, R. (1968). Voltage clamp experiments on frog atrial heart muscle fibres with the sucrose gap technique. Pflügers Arch. 301, 91 - 108.

Rougier, O., Vassort, G., Garnier, D., Gargouil, Y.M. and Coraboeuf, E. (1969). Existence and role of a slow inward current during the frog atrial action potential. Pflügers Arch. 308, 91-110.

Tsien, R.W. (1974a). Effect of epinephine on the pacemaker potassium current of cardiac Purkinje fibres. J. gen. Physiol. (in press).

Tsien, R.W. (1974b). The mode of action of chronotropic agents in cardiac Purkinje fibres. J. gen. Physiol. (in press).

Tsien, R.W., Giles, W.R. and Greengard, P. (1972). Cyclic AMP mediates the action of adrenaline on the action potential plateau of cardiac Purkinje fibres. Nature New Biology. 240, 181-183.

Vassalle, M. (1966). Analysis of cardiac pacemaker potential using a "voltage clamp" technique. Amer. J. Physiol. 210, 1335-1341.

Vassort, G. (1974). Existence of two components in frog cardiac mechanical activity. Influence of Na ions. Europ. J. Cardiol. 1, 163-168.

Weidmann, S. (1951). Effect of current flow on the membrane potential of cardiac muscle. J. Physiol. 115, 227-236.

Weidmann, S. (1955). The effect of the cardiac membrane potential on the rapid availability of the sodium carrying system. _J. Physiol._ 127, 213-214.

Anti-dysrhythmic Drugs—Their Mode of Action

E. M. VAUGHAN WILLIAMS

Department of Pharmacology, Oxford University, U.K.

ANTI-DYSRHYTHMIC DRUGS - THEIR MODE OF ACTION

In some clinical situations the physician may not be interested in the mode of action of the drugs he uses. Provided he can be confident that the remedy will be effective at the dosage administered, he need not concern himself further with such matters, for example, as the biochemical derangements within micro-organisms eliminated. Disorders of cardiac rhythm, however, are so varied, and their causes so little understood, that knowledge of the physiological effects of anti-arrhythmic drugs is a prerequisite for a rational approach to therapy. In the highly developed countries mortality from cardiovascular disease is extremely high. Although there are regional differences, (for example, in Japan cerebral vascular disease predominates, whereas in Europe and the U.S.A. the heart is the primary target) a satisfactory explanation for such variations is not available. What is certain is that vascular deterioration starts early in life and is progressive. Post-mortem examinations performed on battle casualties, accident victims and people meeting other kinds of violent death, have revealed that atheromatous plaques begin to form in the coronaries of quite young persons, in their twenties and thirties. By the age of 50 half the population, even without any symptoms of cardiac disease, have at least one coronary artery occluded by 50% or more, and less than one fifth have entirely unoccluded arteries at this age (Rissanen, 1970). Until about ten years ago fibrillation and severe dysrhythmias were not especially associated with coronary thrombosis, but since the introduction of continuous ECG recording 24 hours a day in intensive care units it has become evident that 95% of patients with cardiac infarction exhibit some episode of dysrhythmias within the first 48 hours (Julian, et al., 1964). One of the most puzzling features of post-mortem examinations of cardiac infarctions was that so many people, especially the younger ones, had died in spite of the fact that the mass of ventricular tissue deprived of its blood supply was often quite small. The implication was that these patients had succumbed to ventricular fibrillation, and that the immediate availability of a really safe and effective anti-dysrhythmic drug could have prolonged a number of lives.

Thus the urgent need for further research into the production of new anti-dysrhythmic compounds can hardly be in doubt. Unfortunately, when one looks for a rational basis upon which a systematic investigation might be founded, the situation is hopelessly confused. There is not even agreement about the classification of the drugs we already have (Vaughan Williams, 1970 ; Bassett and Hoffman, 1971).

Another difficulty impeding the development of new drugs is the lack of a reliable animal model for the study of dysrhythmias. Abnormalities of cardiac rhythm can be produced experimentally by a variety of methods - aconitine, chloroform and adrenaline, acetylcholine and electrical stimulation, overdosage with digitalis, coronary ligation etc. - but such procedures are unreliable and offer no guarantee that results obtained with them are relevant to clinical situations in man. For this reason in recent years the problem has been approached from the opposite end, as it were, and a detailed study has been made of the electrophysiological and other effects of drugs which were known to be anti-dysrhythmic in man, in the hope of finding some accurately measurable common actions. The objective of a search for hard facts about the properties of such agents was twofold. First a screen for new compounds could be designed, because if a new compound also possessed similar properties it would be likely to be anti-dysrhythmic. Secondly, a detailed study of the mode of action of drugs capable of controlling dysrhythmias might throw some light on the cellular basis of the dysrhythmias themselves.

ELECTROPHYSIOLOGY

Before describing the actions of anti-dysrhythmic drugs it may be helpful if I discuss very briefly some current views about the functioning of excitable tissues. It had been known for a couple of generations that the interior of nerves and muscles was negatively charged at rest, the electro-motive force (E) being provided by the relatively high intra-cellular concentration of potassium ions, which could pass more freely out of the cell than the larger negatively charged ions. At one time it was thought that the action potential represented simply a brief short-circuit of this negatively charged potassium battery (E_K), a view supported by the fact that during the action potential the membrane resistance fell. Hodgkin and his colleagues, however, found (Hodgkin, 1958) that during the action potential the inside of nerves actually became <u>positive</u> relative to the outside. Thus there had to be two batteries, not one. They suggested that the second EMF was provided by the concentration difference of sodium ions, high outside, low inside.

At rest this sodium battery (E_{Na}) remained switched off, as it were, but activation was associated with a large increase in sodium permeability, so that a positive charge of sodium ions entered the cell. This action was very brief, lasting less than a millisecond, after which the sodium permeability was inactivated, and the Na-battery switched off again. The importance of this inactivation of sodium permeability was that the membrane would remain absolutely refractory to the passage of further sodium currents until the processes just described had been reversed by repolarization. This may be illustrated by reference to an actual cardiac action potential (Fig.1).

The refractory period in cardiac muscle is extremely long, because repolarization is about 100 times slower than depolarization. In order to measure the rate of depolarization, therefore, it is necessary to look at the intracellularly recorded potentials at a faster sweep speed. The process of activation or depolarization has three phases. At rest (Inside potential negative) sodium permeability is low, as though a gate in the membrane (labelled m) were closed. When current from a neighbouring active region depolarizes a fibre (phase 1), something occurs in the membrane so that permeability to sodium increases (the m-gate opens) and in phase 2 the fibre itself becomes actively depolarized, and begins passively to depolarize the next fibre so that the action potential propagates. Finally (phase 3) the sodium permeability is inactivated,

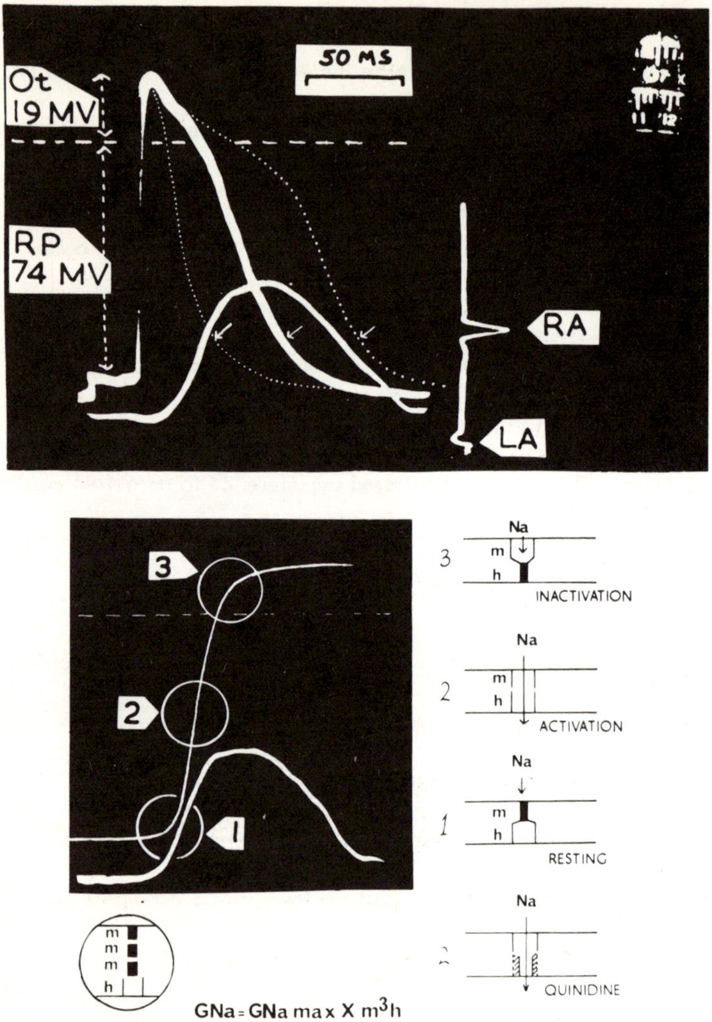

Fig. l. Cardiac action potential. Upper panel. Dashed line: zero potential with electrode outside fibre. Centre trace: electrode inside single cardiac cell showing resting potential (RP) -74 mV. The stimulus in a distant fibre on the left atrium appears as an

(cont.)

(Legend of Fig. I cont.)

artefact. When the active region reaches the cell in which the electrode is situated the inside becomes positive (overshoot, Ot) by +19mV and slowly repolarizes. The arrows indicate the point of repolarization at which a second response would be possible, and the dotted lines indicate that any drug or condition which accelerated or delayed repolarization would shorten or lengthen the absolute refractory period. Vertical trace, right: externally recorded action potentials from left (LA) and right (RA) atrium from which conduction velocity may be calculated. Bottom trace: contraction. Lower panel. Intracellular record at a faster sweep speed. (1) Current flowing into approaching active region begins to depolarize fibre; right: at the resting potential the h gate is open, the m gate closed. (2) Depolarization opens the m gate. Na current into the fibre is maximal. (3) Depolarization has closed the h gate, and Na current is inactivated. Bottom right. The action of quinidine may be to prevent the h gate re-opening fully after repolarization, so that in stage 2 of a depolarization maximum Na current is not reached. Bottom left. If the symbols m and h are the fractions of maximum Na current each gate will pass, and if three m gates are in series with one h gate, the sodium conductance (GNa) at any instant is given by $GNa = GNa\ (maximum)\ m^3h$.

as though another gate (labelled h), in series with the first, became closed. The membrane will thus remain absolutely refractory to sodium current until repolarization has made it possible for the h-gate to re-open. It is at once apparent that any drug or condition which shortened the duration of the cardiac action potential would automatically shorten the refractory period, and so increase the probability of fibrillation. This is, in fact, the effect of acetylcholine, of hypoxia and of halogen anaesthetics, all known to be liable to precipitate dysrhythmias. Conversely, if repolarization were delayed, the refractory period would be prolonged.

So much for the introductory electrophysiology. We may now turn to the actual effects of the drugs themselves.

PHARMACOLOGY

Class 1 Action

In the last few years my colleagues and I have analysed the electrophysiological and other actions of several recently introduced and also of some familiar anti-dysrhythmic compounds, in the hope of arriving at some rational basis for assessment. We have concluded that there are certainly three and possibly four classes of anti-dysrhythmic action. Several drugs have more than one mode of action, and some confusion might have been avoided if a quantitative estimate had been available of the relative concentrations required to produce the respective effects.

Quinidine is the prototype of anti-dysrhythmic drugs and its electrophysiological effects on heart muscle may be considered the first class of anti-dysrhythmic action (Fig.2).

Quinidine caused no change in the resting potential and thus presumably does not interfere with the metabolic processes responsible for ion-pumping across the membrane, so that the potassium battery remains fully charged (Vaughan Williams, 1958). The intracellular concentration of potassium is not lowered by quinidine, nor is the intracellular sodium concentration raised (Goodford and Vaughan Williams, 1962). Nevertheless the maximum rate of depolarization (MRD) was greatly reduced in the presence of quinidine, in spite of the fact that the driving force for depolarization (the voltage of the sodium battery, E_{Na}) was unaffected. It must be assumed, therefore, that quinidine had some <u>direct effect on the membrane</u>, restricting the entry of depolarizing current, as though it were obstructing the full opening of one of the "gates" (see Fig.1, bottom right).

One might ask why should a drug which reduces the rate of entry of depolarizing current be antifibrillatory? It has been known for a long time that, owing to the process of accommodation in excitable tissues, very slowly rising currents fail to excite. Thus, a minimum rate of depolarization must be achieved in order for an action potential to be propagated. It has already been mentioned that repolarization has to

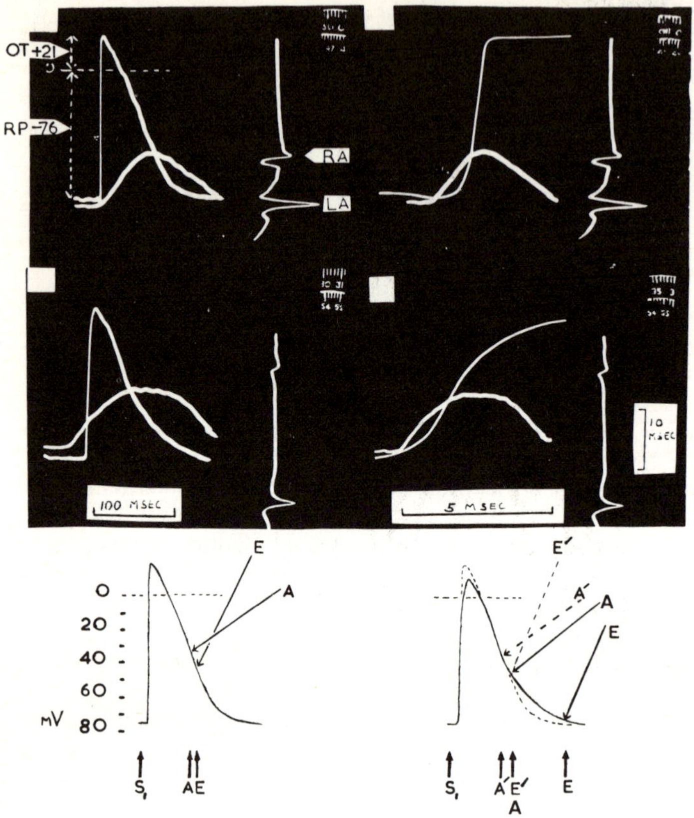

Fig. 2. Effect of quinidine on cardiac intracellular potentials. Upper records: intracellular potentials at slow (left) and fast (right) sweep speeds. Contractions, (below and externally recorded action potentials (vertical traces) are also shown. Lower records. Effect of quinidine, 9 mg/1. Left: There is no change in resting potential, and the tail of repolarization is slightly prolonged. The contraction is dispersed in time, but not reduced, and the conduction velocity

occur before the h-gate can re-open and permit the entry of Na for a second action potential. The effective refractory period may be defined as the point at which the h-gate has opened sufficiently for the rate of rise of a second spike to be fast enough for propagation along the whole muscle to occur. The absolute refractory period is a little shorter

---

is greatly slowed. Right: The maximum rate of depolarization (MRD) is much slower. Diagram. Left: tracing of control intracellular record. At the point of departure of the arrow A, repolarization has proceeded sufficiently far for the h gate to open to an extent which would permit a rate of depolarization sufficient to cause a local, but not a propagated response (absolute refractory period). At the point of departure of E, the h gate has opened further and a stimulus at this point would cause a rate of depolarization fast enough for propagation (effective refractory period). Right: in the presence of quinidine, although the duration of repolarization itself is little affected, direct interference with the mechanism of depolarization makes it necessary for repolarization to proceed much further before a stimulus will cause a rate of depolarization sufficient to permit propagation. Thus the effective refractory period is prolonged, although the absolute refractory period is little changed. The dotted lines are the superimposed controls.

than this, because a stimulus may produce a local response, even though the rate of rise is not fast enough for propagation (see Fig.2, bottom left). In the presence of quinidine and other class 1 drugs the entry of depolarizing current is restricted, and repolarization has, therefore, to proceed much further before the gates can be opened wide enough for the minimum rate of rise for propagation to be reached. Thus the effective refractory period is prolonged by quinidine even though the duration of the action potential itself is not. It was shown in 1958 (Vaughan Williams, 1958) that quinidine reduced the rate of rise of the action potential much more at high than at low frequencies of stimulation. It is thus antifibrillatory because it cuts out the propagation of the abnormal high frequency impulses, but not of the normal mower frequency sinus rhythm.

Quinidine, and other similarly acting compounds are also local anaesthetics on nerve but it must be emphasized that the concentration of the anti-dysrhythmic drugs required to depress excitability in the heart is much lower than that required for the local anaesthesia of nerve. Therein lies their value. Quinidine, and other "class 1" drugs with local anaesthetic action, such as procaine, procainamide and lignocaine, also depress cardiac contractions, but usually higher concentrations are required to depress contractions than to reduce the maximum rate of depolarization.

The question must now be considered how lignocaine and

diphenylhydantoin exert their anti-dysrhythmic action. Lignocaine is a well-known local anaesthetic, and one might naturally have supposed that it would act in the same way as procaine or procainamide and other drugs with local anaesthetic properties. It has been suggested, however, in particular by (Davis and Temte, 1969) and (Bigger and Mandel, 1970), that the anti-dysrhythmic actions of lignocaine and DPH are fundamentally different. Although these authors agreed that lignocaine and DPH reduced the maximum rate of depolarization (MRD) of cardiac muscle they claimed that higher concentrations were required to produce the effect that would occur in the blood of treated patients. We noted that the evidence on which this contention was based was obtained from tissues bathed with solutions very low in potassium. We have re-investigated the electrophysiological effects of lignocaine and DPH both in low and in normal potassium solutions, and so far as the experimental observations are concerned, we have fully confirmed the findings of Bigger and his colleagues. At abnormally low potassium concentrations, higher concentrations of the drugs are needed to depress MRD. At a normal potassium concentration, however, both lignocaine and DPH depress MRD at concentrations well within the range found clinically (Fig. 3).

We have concluded, therefore, that lignocaine and DPH are probably anti-dysrhythmic because they depress MRD in common with

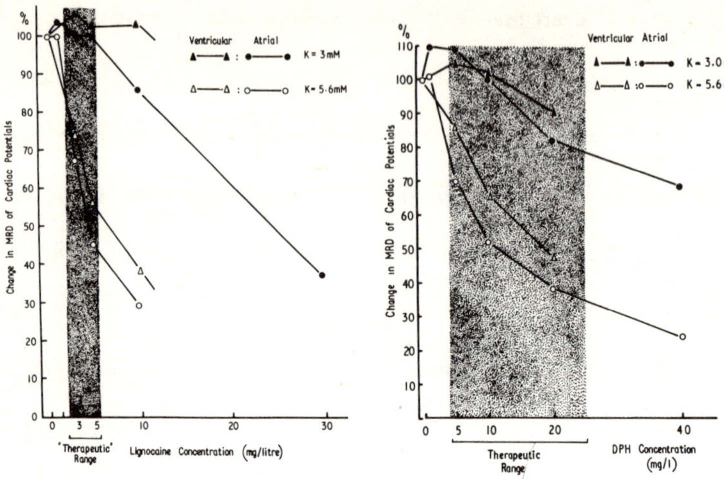

Fig. 3. Effect of lignocaine and diphenylhydantoin on the maximum rate of depolarization (MRD) of cardiac muscle in normal and low external K concentration. Ordinates: % reduction in MRD from controls (the control MRD is faster in low K than in normal K). Stippled areas indicate the range of concentrations of the drugs actually observed in the serum of successfully treated patients. Low potassium shifts the dose-response curves to the right, with the implication that a fall in serum K would prevent a patient responding to the drugs.

other local anaesthetic type drugs (Singh and Vaughan Williams, 1971). I would like to emphasize, however, that this is not to claim there are no differences between the actions of, say, quinidine and lignocaine in man or whole animals. On the contrary, there are several, especially in relation to their negative inotropic action, to their duration of action, to their atropine-like properties and to their effects on the central nervous system. So far as their direct effect on the cardiac membrane itself is concerned, however, there seems to be no reason to suppose that their mode of action is fundamentally different. We confirmed that low potassium caused a shift in the dose response curve and this explains the fact that lignocaine is ineffective in patients with low serum potassium (Pamintuan et al., 1970).

Class 2 Action

It is well known that hyperactivity of the sympathetic system is liable to induce dysrhythmias and we may now turn to the second class of anti-dysrhythmic action, exhibited by drugs with antisympathetic effects, either by β-receptor blockade, or by interference with the release of sympathetic transmitters (bretylium, guanethidine). Such antisympathetic drugs would naturally be expected to be most effective in dysrhythmias associated with excessive sympathetic drive, but we found (Vaughan Williams and Sekiya, 1963) that β-receptor blocking drugs protected against ouabain-induced fibrillation also. This was in agreement with the finding of (Mendez et al., 1961) that deprivation of sympathetic drive by sympathectomy and adrenalectomy prevented the occurrence of ventricular fibrillation after digitalis in dogs.

We soon discovered, however, that pronethalol and propranolol, and several other β-receptor blocking compounds, were powerful local anaesthetics, more potent than procaine. They also reduced the rate of rise of the action potential, as did the other anti-dysrhythmic drugs with local anaesthetic properties.

The question arose, therefore, whether β-receptor blockade had anything to do with the protection against digitalis, and some authors maintained that this action ("quinidine-like' or 'class 1") was sufficient to account for the prevention of digitalis-induced dysrhythmias. The laevo-isomer of propranolol, however, which has the same local anaesthetic potency as the dextro-isomer but is 100 times more active as a β-receptor blocker, was much more effective than the dextro-isomer in protecting against ouabain-induced ventricular fibrillation. There is much further recent evidence in favour of the original contention that antisympathetic drugs protect not only against dysrhythmias associated with excess sympathetic activity but also against those occurring after coronary ligation or digitalis intoxication (Dohadwalla et al., 1969). Further support for this view is provided by the effect of bretylium (Fig.4). This drug blocks the release of noradrenaline from sympathetic nerve endings. It was also found to protect guinea pigs against ouabain-induced ventricular fibrillation (Papp and Vaughan Williams, 1969). When we looked at its electrophysiological properties however, we found that it had no "class 1" or direct membrane properties whatev

It is thus apparent that drugs with an antisympathetic action, whether produced by neurone blockade or by competition for transmitter at receptors, are anti-dysrhythmic in their own right, as it were. The removal of sympathetic background reduces the probability of dysrhythmia, whatever the precipitating factor may be.

Class 3 Action

In the hope of finding a lead for the development of new anti-dysrhythmic drugs, it was thought worthwhile to investigate the electro-physiological effects of conditions known to be associated with dysrhythmias. Hypoxia and halogen anaesthetics have already been mentioned. Now it is well established that hyperthyroidism causes atrial fibrillation, whereas in myxoedema, cardiac irregularities, apart from an occasional extrasystole associated with very low heart rates, are extremely rare. We have investigated the effects on cardiac intracellular potentials of hyper- and hypothyroidism. It was thought possible, for example, that in hypothyroidism, the rate of rise of the action potential might be reduced. It is known that in myxoedema the electrocardiogram is of low voltage, and it was a reasonable guess that the reduced metabolic rate might have interfered in some way with the ionic pumps, so that the voltages of the sodium and potassium batteries could have been reduced. Actual experiment indicated, however, that this was not the case (Freedberg et al., 1970) (Fig. 5).

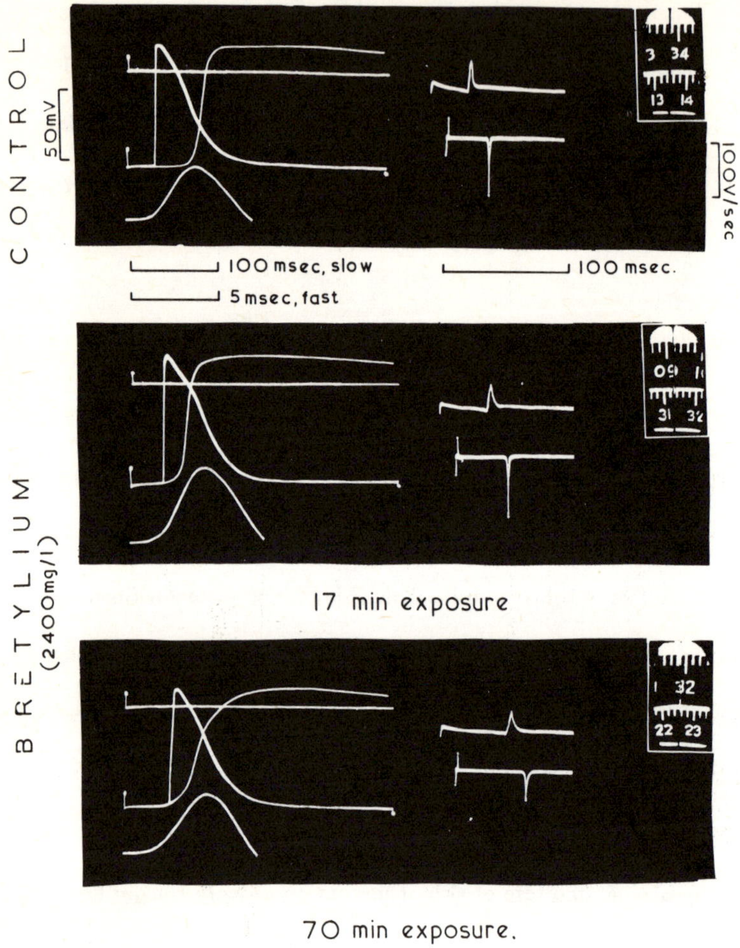

Fig. 4. The effect of bretylium on cardiac intracellular potentials. In each panel: Left: horizontal trace = zero potential; middle traces = intracellularly recorded potentials at slow and fast sweep speeds, superimposed; lower traces = contractions. Right. Upper trace: stimulus artefact from electrode on left atrium, and

Evidently alterations of thyroid state had no effect upon the resting or action potential voltages, nor was there any effect of significance on the rate of rise of the action potential. Presumably the low ECG voltage observed in myxoedema is due to some factor such as the presence of interstitial fluid or pericardial effusion. Differences in thyroid state did have, however, a very big influence on the duration of the action potential (Fig. 6 and 7).

We thus seemed to have hit upon a third way in which an anti-dysrhythmic effect might be achieved, if a drug could be found, which, without being generally antithyroid, might nevertheless imitate the effects of hypothyroidism on cardiac muscle.

The anti-anginal drug Amiodarone has been in use for many years, and its general pharmacological properties have been extensively studied by Charlier et al., 1968). Our own investigations showed that this drug

---

externally recorded action potential from external electrode on right atrium, for measurement of conduction velocity. Lower trace: differentiated record (dV/dt) of the intracellular trace. The depth of the spike is proportional to MRD. Bretylium, even at a concentration of 20 mg/1, had no direct "class 1" depressant effect on the cardiac membrane.

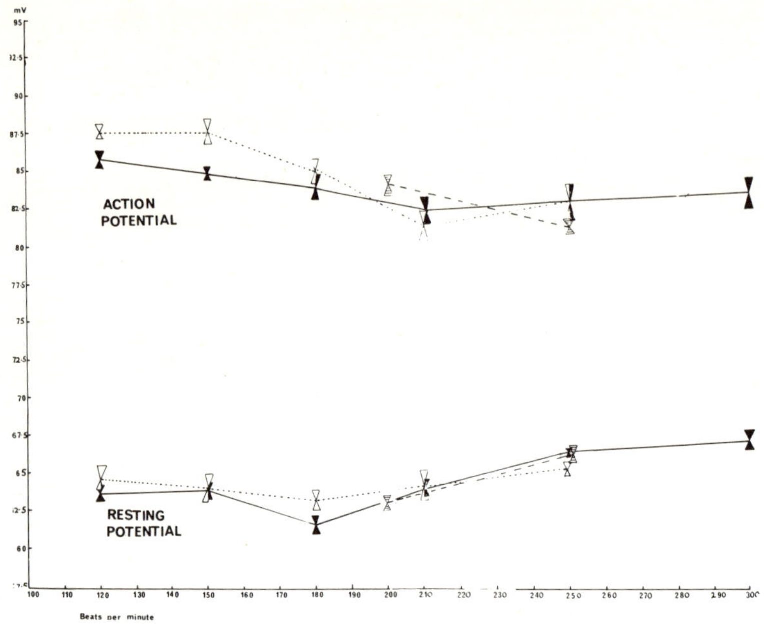

Fig. 5. Intracellularly recorded resting and action potentials of rabbit atria in different thyroid states. To avoid errors which might be introduced by differences of spontaneous heart rate, the measurements were made in atria electrically stimulated over a wide range of frequencies. Ordinate: millivolts. Abscissa: driving frequency, beats per min. Controls: black triangles and solid line. Hypothyroid animals; open triangles and dotted lines. Hyperthyroid animals: striped triangles and dashed line. The apices of the triangles meet at the mean, and the height of each triangle equals the standard error.

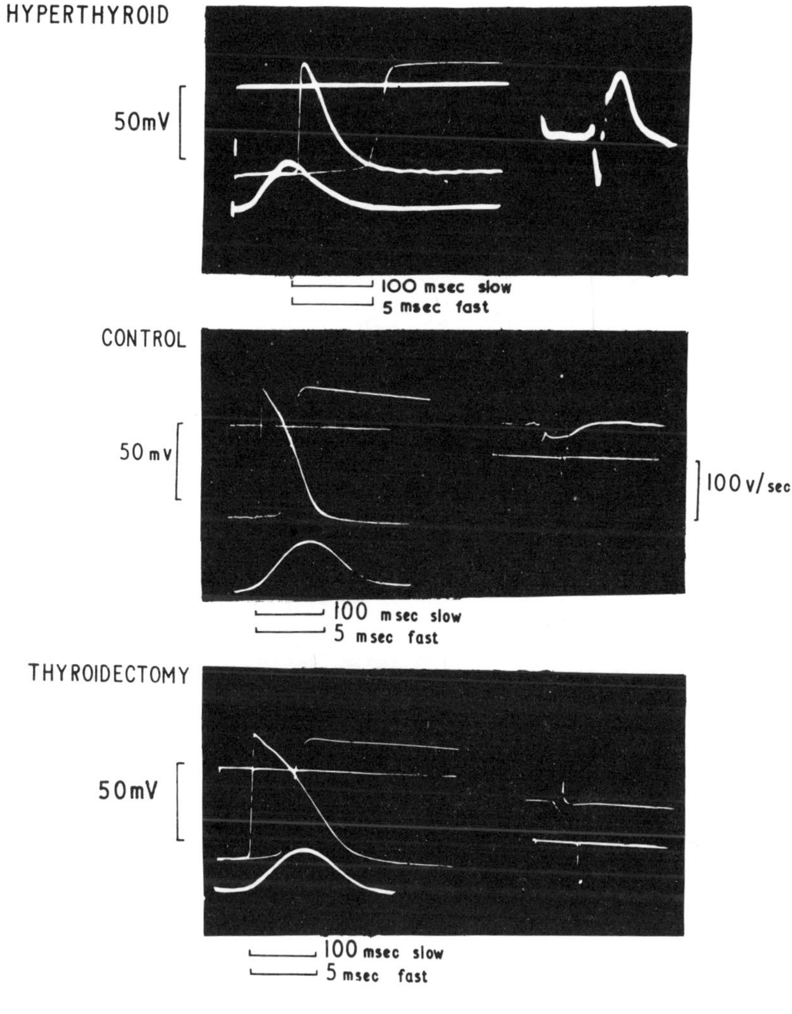

Fig. 6. Description as for Fig. 4. Differences of thyroid state had little effect on resting and action potential voltages, nor on the rate of rise of the potential, but greatly influenced the rate of repolarization.

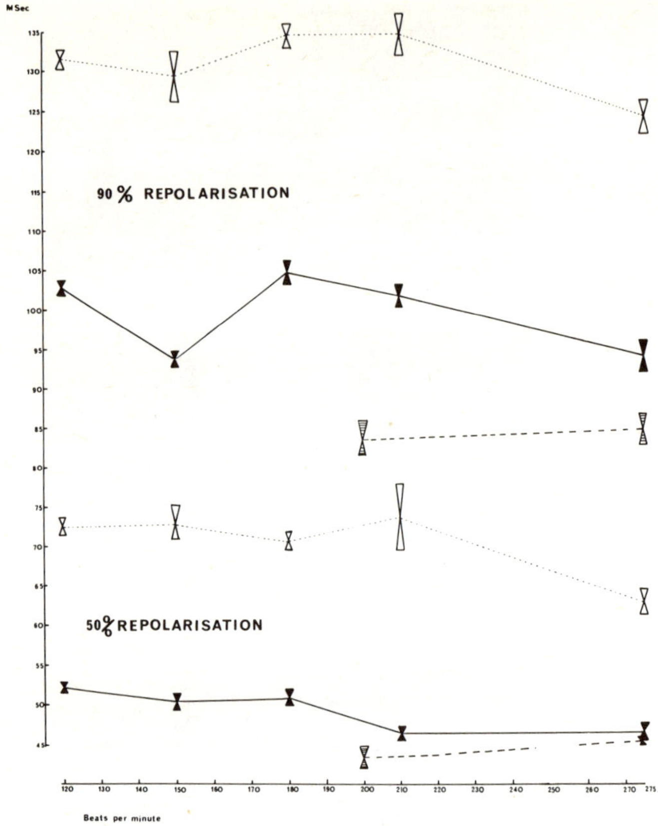

Fig. 7. Duration of action potential from peak to 90% repolarization (upper curves) and to 50% repolarization lower curves. Ordinate: milliseconds. Abscissa: driving frequency, beats per min. Symbols as for Fig. 5.

prolonged the cardiac action potential, as did thyroidectomy (Singh and Vaughan Williams, 1970) (Fig. 8).

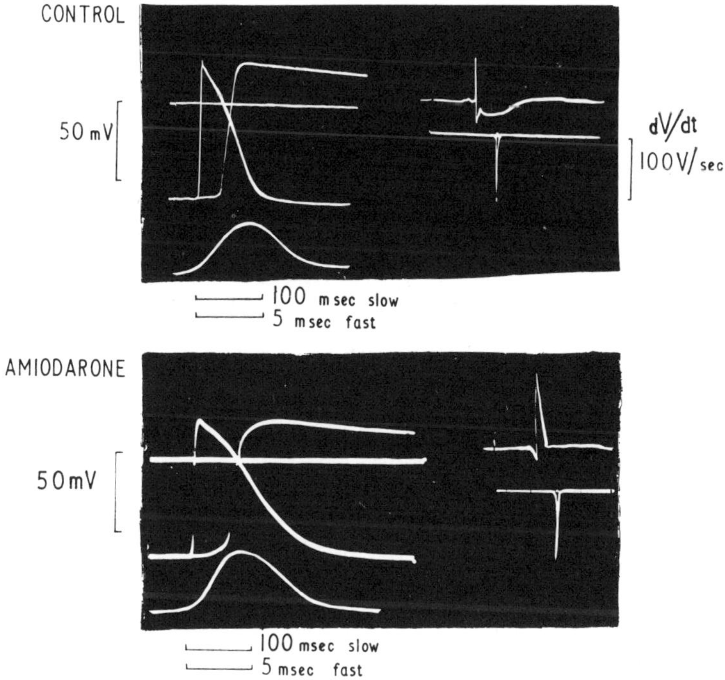

Fig. 8. The effect of amiodarone on atrial intracellular potentials. Description as for Fig. 1. The atria were taken from rabbits given 20 mg/kg amiodarone daily intraperitoneally for 6 weeks. The treatment had no effect on resting or action potential voltages, and only a minor effect on MRD, but greatly prolonged the duration of the action potential.

It must be emphasised, however, that amiodarone is not a general antithyroid drug. It has no effect on the weight of the thyroid gland,

and no signs of hypothyroidism have appeared in patients treated for prolonged periods. Amiodarone is a potent anti-arrhythmic drug in animals and in man (Ferrero and Benabderhamane, 1972).

Class 4 Action

Verapamil (isoptin) is an anti-dysrhythmic drug which does not have any of the above three classes of action (Singh and Vaughan Williams, 1972). It appears to reduce calcium permeability, and the suggestion that this may constitute a fourth class of anti-dysrhythmic action carries with it the interesting implication that inward calcium movement could cause dysrhythmias by carrying depolarizing current in addition to the normal sodium current.

ANTI-DYSRHYTHMIC ACTION. THEORY AND PRACTICE.

Theoretical work with computed models of sheets of simulated cardiac cells has delineated the requirements for the development of re-entry circuits as follows:-

1) The matrix must be of sufficient size (about 10^3 cells).

2) There must be multiple contacts between cells, permitting conduction to emerge from an active cell in several possible alternative directions when it is blocked in others (e.g. a hexagonal honeycomb array permitting each cell a contact with six others).

3) The cells must not all be the same; inhomogeneity in electrical threshold, refractory period etc. must occur in the matrix.

4) The mean absolute refractory period must not be longer than a certain limiting value.

5) There must be an ectopic or out-of-phase stimulus or a high frequency pacemaker.

To what extent can it be shown that suitable conditions exist in reality in mammalian cardiac muscle? First, in man the matrix is certainly much larger than that required; moreover it is 3-dimensional, whereas the models are only 2-dimensional (Moe et al., 1964). Secondly, the electron microscope has revealed that each cell makes contact with perhaps as many as six neighbours, certainly with several. Inhomogeneity of electrical activity of different regions of cardiac muscle has been demonstrated experimentally, so that the third criterion is also fulfilled (Sano et al., 1959; Han and Moe, 1964). As to the fourth, the greater probability of dysrhythmias associated with a short action potential has already been noted, whereas in hypothyroidism rarity of dysrhythmia is associated with a long one. Similar findings have been confirmed in man (Olsson et al., 1971; Cotoi et al., 1972). Finally, sources of ectopic activation are a common feature of numerous pathological cardiac states, and the importance of parasystolic pacemakers in the aetiology of many kinds of human dysrhythmias has been emphasised by (Schamroth, 1971) in a recent review.

How, then, may the classes of anti-dysrhythmic action described above be related to the theoretical considerations concerning the cellular basis of cardiac dysrhythmias? The class 2 (antisympathetic) action can remove or retard parasystolic pacemaking sources activated by excessive sympathetic activity or by circulating catecholamines. The third class of action, by prolonging the cardiac action potential, would push the absolute refractory period beyond the limiting value. The first class of action would directly impede cell to cell conduction at a high frequency. Thus the analysis of anti-dysrhythmic action into the first three classes described above does fit rather well theories concerning the cellular basis of cardiac dysrhythmias. As to the fourth class, the role of calcium in the cardiac action potential is still too uncertain to permit profitable speculation.

Even if the classification of anti-dysrhythmic drugs outlined above, and its relevance to models of dysrhythmias, were accepted, the physician might still wonder whether he is any nearer, in practical terms, to a rational approach to the treatment of clinically encountered abnormalities of cardiac rhythm.

Clearly the problem of treatment is greatly simplified if a dysrhythmia is primary and there is no evidence of myocardial degeneration or cardiac vascular disease. In a post-menopausal woman, for example, whose tachycardia is largely caused or exacerbated by anxiety, exhibition of a class 2 antisympathetic drug would be rational therapy, and a beta-receptor blocker provides adequate control in doses too small to present any danger. The same applies to other stress induced dysrhythmias, as during induction of anaesthesia (Payne and Senfield, 1964) or such occupations as skiing, flying, driving, public speaking etc. (Taggart et al., 1969). In such circumstances the choice of any particular β-blocking drug is probably of little importance.

Atrial fibrillation can usually be corrected by D.C. shock, but maintenance in sinus rhythm remains a problem. Patients who relapse into fibrillation have shorter than normal action potentials, and exhibition of a drug with a class 3 action, prolonging the duration of the action potential, would be appropriate. Amiodarone and oxyfedrine both have such an action on prolonged treatment.

When a dysrhythmia is a manifestation of serious cardiac disease, however, control is more difficult and dangerous, and even though correction of the abnormal rhythm may prolong life, it does not, of course, remove the underlying pathology. After cardiac infarction dysrhythmias occur in 90% or more of patients (Julian et al., 1964). Factors increasing the probability of re-entry are the shortening of action potentials in hypoxic fibres, and inhomogeneity of conduction pathways through and around damaged areas. In addition, the level of circulating catecholamines is extremely high (Valori et al., 1967) and has been correlated with the incidence of rhythm abnormalities.

In these circumstances also, therefore, exhibition of a β-blocker would be rational therapy, but brings with it the danger that an ailing myocardium deprived of its sympathetic drive may fail altogether. What is needed is a drug which could block receptors mediating chronotropic effects without blocking those mediating inotropic effects, but no such compound is yet available. In its absence, extreme caution is necessary, so that a level of blockade is selected which eliminates the excessive adrenergic stimulation facilitating the development of dysrhythmias, but which is not so complete that inotropic drive is endangered. The choice of drug may be important, and in this context three considerations are relevant.

1) It has been suggested that β-receptor blocking drugs which have some partial agonist (sympathomimetic) activity of their own may be preferable (e.g. alprenolol). The logic of this is not apparent, however. Why should the activity of a partial agonist be preferable to that of noradrenaline and adrenaline, themselves the natural transmitters? If agonist activity is required, it should be sufficient to reduce the degree of blockade.

2) Some β-blockers have class 1 activity as well (notably propranolol, alprenolol and oxprenolol) (Morales-Aguilera and Vaughan Williams, 1965 ; Singh and Vaughan Williams, 1970) and it has been suggested that this "non-specific" depressant activity may be

associated with a negative inotropic action. If this were so, practolol and pindolol (LB 46) would be advantageous (Singh and Vaughan Williams, 1971) but no satisfactory evidence is available that the liability of β-blockers to precipitate failure is in fact related to any direct negative inotropic action. Some class 1 drugs, reducing MRD in cardiac muscle and with local anaesthetic properties, increase myocardial contractions (Vaughan Williams and Szekeres, 1961; Bagwell et al., 1973).

3) Some β-receptor blocking drugs are more active in blocking peripheral receptors, mediating vasodilatation in the limbs, than in blocking cardiac receptors. Among such drugs are pindolol and propranolol, and the compounds with substituents at position 2 of the ring, alprenolol and oxprenolol (Singh and Vaughan Williams, 1970). These compounds, against a background of circulating catecholamines, are actually hypertensive. It is possible, therefore, that such β-blockers could, in the presence of high circulating catecholamines, cause a rise in peripheral resistance which could throw an additional load on the myocardium. If this is so, a cardioselective β-receptor blocking drug, such as practolol, would have an advantage. One of the features conferring cardioselectivity is substitution on position 4 of the ring (Vaughan Williams et al., 1973), and doubtless new compounds even more cardioselective than practolol will eventually be available.

Which, if any, of the above considerations is important will have to be determined by further research.

Diminution of sympathetic background removes only one of the factors increasing the probability of dysrhythmias, and when this is insufficient recourse to a drug with a class 1 action is necessary. If exhibition of such compounds (lignocaine, procaineamide, diphenyldantoin, quinidine) is still ineffective, an obvious precaution is to measure the serum potassium level, and if this is low, to correct it. Theoretically, it would seem justifiable to raise the serum potassium above normal, in order to increase the efficacy of the drug, but here again further research is required to determine how far this would be a safe procedure.

Finally, in the future, it is probable that drugs with an acute class 3 action will become available. At present the only drugs with such an acute action, INPEA and sotalol (Singh and Vaughan Williams, 1971 ; Singh and Vaughan Williams, 1970), are also β-blockers, and the class 3 action would be accompanied by further β-blockade. Amiodarone and oxyfedrine require prolonged administration to produce this effect.

In conclusion, it is apparent that so far there is no established procedure, authenticated by experimental evidence, the progressive application of which would ensure the optimum utilization of currently available drugs to correct dysrhythmias in gravely ill patients. On the other hand, a great deal is known of the electrophysiological and pharmacological properties of the individual compounds, so that the research from which such a procedure may emerge can at least now be planned on a rational basis.

REFERENCES

Bagwell, E.E., Polster, P. and Vaughan Williams, E.M. (1973). The effects on cardiac muscle and nerve of a fluorinated decahydroquinoline derivative, L7810, rapidly absorbed after oral administration. Brit. J. Pharmacol. 48, 183-193.

Bassett, A.L. and Hoffman, B.F. (1971). Antiarrhythmic drugs: electrophysiological actions. Ann. Rev. Pharmac. 11, 143-170.

Bigger, J.T. and Mandel, W.J. (1970). Effect of lidocaine on the electrophysiological properties of ventricular muscle and purkinje fibers. J. Clin. Invest. 49, 63-77.

Charlier, R., Deltour, G., Baudine, A. and Chaillet, F. (1968). Pharmacology of amiodarone, and anti-anginal drug with a new biological profile. Arzneimittelforsch. 18, 1408-1417.

Cotoi, S., Constantinescu, L. and Gavrilescu, S. (1972). The effect of thyroid state on manophasic action potential in human heart. Experientia, 28, 797-798.

Davis, L.D. and Temte, J.V. (1969). Electrophysiological actions of lidocaine on canine ventricular muscle and purkinje fibers. Circ. Res. 24, 639-655.

Dohadwalla, A.N., Freedberg, A.S. and Vaughan Williams, E.M. (1969). The relevance of beta-receptor blockade to ouabain-induced cardiac arrhythmias. Brit. J. Pharmacol. 36, 257-267.

Ferrero, C. and Benabderhamane, M. (1972). Terapia medica del flutter atriale. Giorn. It. Card. 2, 186.

Freedberg, A.S., Papp, I. Gy. and Vaughan Williams, E.M. (1970). The effect of altered thyroid state on atrial intracellular potentials. J. Physiol. 207, 357-369.

Goodford, P.J. and Vaughan Williams, E.M. (1962). Intracellular Na and K concentrations of rabbit atria, in relation to the action of quinidine. J. Physiol. 160, 483-493.

Han, J. and Moe, G.K. (1964). Nonuniform recovery of excitability in ventricular muscle. Circ. Res. 14, 44-60.

Hodgkin, A.L. (1958). Ionic movements and electrical activity in giant nerve fibers. Proc. Roy. Soc. B. 148, 1-37.

Julian, D.G., Valentine, P.A. and Miller, G.G. (1964). Disturbances of rate, rhythm and conduction in acute myocardial infarction: a prospective study of 100 consecutive unselected patients with the aid of electrocardiographic monitoring. Amer. J. Med. 37, 915-927.

Mendez, C., Aceves, J. and Mendez, R. (1961). Inhibition of adrenergic cardiac acceleration by cardiac glycosides. J. Pharmacol. Exp. Ther. 131, 199-204.

Moe, G.K., Rheinboldt, W.C. and Abildskov, S.A. (1964). A computer model of atrial fibrillation. Amer. Heart J. 67, 200-220.

Morales-Aguilera, A. and Vaughan Williams, E.M. (1965). The effects of cardiac muscle of beta-receptor antagonists in relation to their activity as local anaesthetics. Brit. J. Pharmacol. 24, 332-338.

Olsson, S.B., Cotoi, S. and Varnauskas, E. (1971). Monophasic action potential and sinus rhythm stability after conversion of atrial fibrillation. Acta Med. Scand. 190, 381-387.

Pamintuan, J.C., Dreifus, L.S. and Watanabe, Y. (1970). Comparative mechanisms of antiarrhythmic agents. Amer. J. Cardiol. 26, 512-519.

Papp, J. Gy. and Vaughan Williams, E.M. (1969). The effect of bretylium on intracellular cardiac action potentials in relation to its antiarrhythmic and local anaesthetic activity. Brit. J. Pharmacol. 37, 380-390.

Payne, J.P. and Senfield, R.M. (1964). Pronethalol in treatment of ventricular arrhythmias during anaesthesia. Brit. Med. J. (i), 603-604.

Rissanen, V.T. (1970). Occurrence of coronary occlusions in cases of coronary death and accidental death. Adv. Cardiol. 4, 99-111.

Sano, T., Takayama, N. and Shimamoto, T. (1959). Directional difference of conduction velocity in the cardiac ventricular syncytium studied by microelectrodes. Circ. Res. 7, 262-267.

Schamroth, L. (1971). The physiological basis of ectopic ventricular rhythm: a unifying concept. South Afr. Med. J. Supplement p3-26. Vol. 45.

Singh, B.N. and Vaughan Williams, E.M. (1970). Local anaesthetic and antiarrhythmic actions of alprenolol relative to its effect on intracellular potentials and other properties of isolated cardiac muscle. Brit. J. Pharmacol. 38, 749-757.

Singh, B.N. and Vaughan Williams, E.M. (1970). The effect of amiodarone, a new anti-anginal drug, on cardiac muscle. Brit. J. Pharmacol. 39, 657-667.

Singh, B.N. and Vaughan Williams, E.M. (1970). A third class of antiarrhythmic action. Effects on atrial and ventricular intracellular potentials, and other pharmacological actions on cardiac muscle, MJ 1999 and AH 3474. Brit. J. Pharmacol. 39, 675-687.

Singh, B.N. and Vaughan Williams, E.M. (1971). Effects on cardiac muscle of the adrenoceptor blocking drugs IMPEA and LB46 in relation to their local anaesthetic action on nerve. Brit. J. Pharmacol. 43, 10-22.

Singh, B.N. and Vaughan Williams, E.M. (1971). Effect of altering potassium concentration on the action of lidocaine and diphenylhydantoin on rabbit atrial and ventricular muscle. Circ. Res. 29, 286-295.

Singh, B.N. and Vaughan Williams, E.M. (1972). A fourth class of antidysrhythmic action? Effect of verapamil on ouabain toxicity, on atrial and ventricular intracellular potentials, and on other features of cardiac function. Cardiovasc. Res. 6, 109-119.

Taggart, P., Gibbons, D. and Somerville, W. (1969). Some effects of motor-car driving on the normal and abnormal heart. Brit. Med. J. 4, 130-134.

Valori, C., Thomas, M. and Shillingford, J.P. (1967). Urinary excretion of free noradrenaline and adrenaline following acute myocardial infarction. Lancet 1, 127-130.

Vaughan Williams, E.M. (1958). The mode of action of quinidine on isolated rabbit atria interpreted from intracellular potential records. Brit. J. Pharmacol. 13, 276-286.

Vaughan Williams, E.M. (1970). Classification of antiarrhythmic drugs. Symposium on Cardiac Arrhythmias (E. Sandoe, E. Flensted-Jensen and K.H. Olesen, eds) pp.449-472. AB Astra, Sodertalje, Sweden.

Vaughan Williams, E.M., Bagwell, E.E. and Singh, B.N. (1973). Cardiospecificity of receptor blockade. A comparison of the relative potencies on cardiac and peripheral vascular adrenoceptors of propranolol, of practolol and its ortho-substituted isomer, and of oxprenolol and its para-substituted isomer. Cardiovasc. Res. 7, 226-240.

Vaughan Williams, E.M., and Sekiya, A. (1963). Prevention of arrhythmias due to cardiac glycosides by block of sympathetic B receptors. Lancet (i), 420-421.

Vaughan Williams, E.M. and Szekeres, L. (1961). A comparison of tests for antifibrillatory action. Brit. J. Pharmacol. 17, 424-432.

Beta-adrenoceptor Blockade

A. M. BARRETT

Department of Pharmacology, University of Leeds, U.K.

INTRODUCTION

In considering the ways in which β-adrenoceptor antagonists achieve their clinical effects, two important and related points merit general attention. First, the wide range of physiological functions influenced by the sympathetic division of the autonomic nervous system provides the fundamental basis on which the apparently diverse clinical applications of β-blocking therapy are made. In other words the observation of clinical benefit in a particular condition following the administration of a β-adrenoceptor antagonist has sometimes revealed a previously unsuspected sympathetic component e.g. in the management of heroin addicts (Grosz, 1972) or migraine (Wideroe and Vigander, 1974). Second, virtually all chemical substances exerting a therapeutic action exhibit a dose-related effect. The majority of clinical evaluations of new drugs attempt to establish a difference between the new agent and placebo treatment which achieves statistical significance. This is quite different from establishing the dose producing maximal clinical benefit for a drug of proven clinical efficacy. There is usually a substantial difference between threshold and maximal effect dose levels. It is perhaps significant that the two clinical investigators (Prichard and Zacharias) most frequently associated with "high doses" of β-blocking drugs are most concerned with attainment of maximal benefit and are wholly familiar with the nature of the pharmacological dose-response curve e.g. Gillam and Prichard, 1971 (see Fig. 6).

Cardiac function is modulated continuously by the autonomic nervous system, the heart receiving fibres from both sympathetic and parasympathetic sources. From the onset, it is important to appreciate the dual nature of this control mechanism. Whereas sympathetic stimulation augments cardiac activity, vagal stimulation decreases it. Reduction or elimination of either system exposes the heart to the unchecked influence of the other. For example, vagal section leads to cardiac acceleration, partly due to loss of inhibitory effects and partly to unopposed sympathetic influence. Conversely thoracic sympathectomy is followed by slowing of the heart mainly due to unopposed vagal action.

There are five principal areas of cardiovascular disease in which β-adrenoceptor antagonists may be used with advantage

1) Irregularities of cardiac rhythm
2) Angina pectoris
3) Hypertension
4) Hypertrophic sub-aortic stenosis
5) Miscellaneous - including thyrotoxicosis, phaeochromocytoma, tetralogy of Fallot and hyperkinetic syndromes.

In all of these situations, clinical benefit can be traced to the primary pharmacological action of the β-adrenoceptor antagonists i.e. selective sympathoplegia.

Transference of nervous impulses to innervated organ is effected by a chemical substance released from the nerve terminals. For sympathetic autonomic nerves the agent is noradrenaline. Under certain conditions the release of adrenaline from the adrenal medulla into the systemic circulation may re-inforce the transmitter action. Noradrenaline reacts in some way with a specific part of the cellular structure where it induces a chain of biochemical events resulting in the development of an observable response e.g. a rise in peripheral resistance. The specific attachment site is termed a receptor, in this case an adrenoceptor (Fig. 1). Pharmacological receptors can not be identified in physical

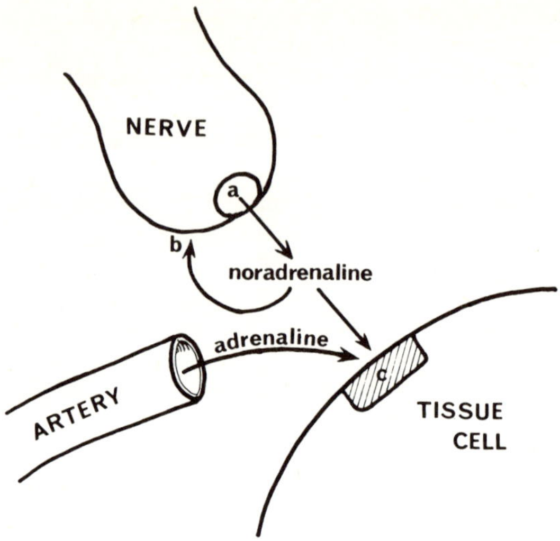

Figure 1.

Diagrammatic representation of a sympathetic neuroeffector junction, showing (a) storage vesicle from which noradrenaline is released on neural stimulation; (b) site of active re-uptake of released transmitter; and (c) specific attachment site or adrenoceptor on tissue cell responding to sympathetic activation.

terms nor can they be visualized or isolated chemically. They remain part of a working concept but there is powerful evidence to support it.

a) biological responses are often remarkably selective rather than general throughout an organism.

b) responses occur to minute concentrations of active agent

(for example, Clark (1933) calculated that an effective concentration of acetylcholine on frog heart would only cover one 6000th of the surface area of individual responding ventricular cells.).

c) quantitative treatment of the reaction between an active agent and the "receptor molecule" shows a reasonable fit to the Michaelis-Menten kinetic equations for enzymic interactions (Jenkinson, 1960).

d) minor modification of the chemistry of an active molecule leads to a dramatic lowering potency

e) when the active molecule is asymmetrical, one isomeric configuration is significantly more active than the other

f) selective antagonists are known which will cancel the actions of one active agent without modification of the responses to others.

From such evidence we derive the belief that pharmacological receptors consist of a specialized surface, containing specific chemical groups in some particular spatial arrangement, so that only an active molecule with the complementary groups appropriately arranged will be able to react (Paton and Payne, 1968).

Pharmacological analysis suggests that mammalian systems possess two distinct types of adrenoceptor which have been designated quite arbitrarily α- and β-adrenoceptors. In the cardiovascular system adrenoceptors in arterial muscle are of the α- category whereas those in the heart are of the β- category. In addition to these "innervated" adrenoceptors, certain areas of vascular smooth muscle also possess receptors of the β-type where there is no proven connexion between nerve supply and initiation of response. These β-adrenoceptors only respond therefore to reactive circulating substances and not to electrical nerve stimulation. Those chemical substances classified as β-adrenoceptor antagonists have a capacity to occupy β-adrenoceptor sites and thus to deny access to released transmitter substance. They do not occupy α-adrenoceptor sites for which there are distinct alternative antagonists i.e. α-adrenoceptor antagonists (Fig. 2).

In the present context we are principally concerned with β-adrenoceptor sites within the heart itself. The transmitter substance is noradrenaline and its release brings about an increase in most aspects of myocardial performance. There is one common confusing misconception which must be first dispelled. Many clinicians seem to hold the view that noradrenaline lowers the heart rate. That is correct if exogenous material is injected intravenously. But the cause of the bradycardia is vagal slowing as a consequence of the rise in blood pressure. Noradrenaline activates the α-adrenoceptors in vascular muscle and the β-adrenoceptors in the heart but in conscious man the reflex effects predominate. Although it is true that agents other than noradrenaline have greater affinity for β-adrenoceptors, this substance remains the natural transmitter and is indeed

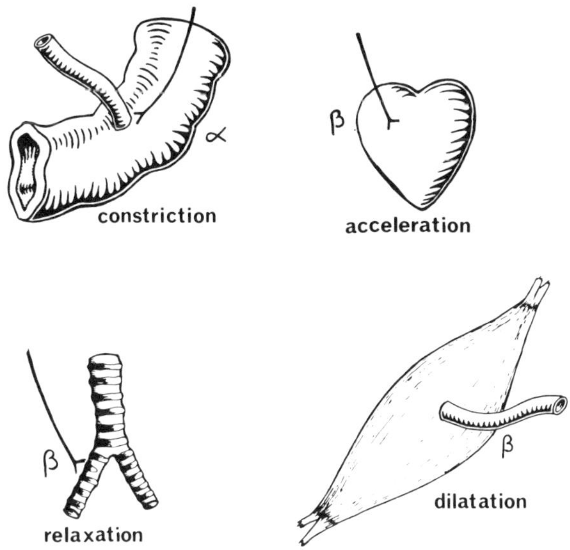

Figure 2.

Diagrammatic representation of distribution of adrenoceptor sub-categories in four tissues indicating nature of response to sympathetic stimulation. Adrenoceptors in arterial muscle of vessels supplying gut, heart and lungs are in close approximation to sympathetic nerve terminals whereas this is not the case for adrenoceptors of the β-category in blood vessels in voluntary muscle. The a-adrenoceptors are blocked by phenoxybenzamine and phentolamine but not by propranolol. The β-adrenoceptors are blocked by propranolol, but not by phenoxybenzamine or phentolamine irrespective of the presence or absence of nerve terminals.

responsible for the dramatic changes in heart rate recorded by our colleagues who give lectures or drive racing cars! (Sommerville, Taggart and Carruthers, 1971; Taggart, Gibbons and Sommerville, 1969). One further point, the antagonism of β-adrenoceptor blocking drugs is not only specific for β-adrenoceptor stimulants, it is also competitive. By this is meant that the definition of "a blocking dose" can only be given in terms of the amount of stimulation at the relevant time. Technically we speak of the dose-response curve being shifted to the left but in practical terms a given degree of inhibition can be overcome by either stepping up the frequency of stimulation or increasing the available amount of stimulating agent (for fuller treatment see Barrett, 1973).

No consideration of the effects of noradrenaline is complete without recognition of the processes which terminate its action at a particular site. Apart from diffusion and loss into extracellular fluid, enzymatic degradation and neuronal uptake are the most important factors. Quantitatively the latter mechanism is of the greatest significance (see Iversen, 1973) when up to 80% of noradrenaline released from nerve terminals may be actively recaptured by the neural tissue. This uptake mechanism is an active process which is sensitive to inhibition. Cocaine and, clinically more importantly, imipramine and its analogues are particularly powerful in this context. The presence of such an inhibitor of noradrenaline uptake will increase the locally available concentration of noradrenaline at the receptor site. Under such circumstances, having in mind the competitive nature of the action of β-blocking drugs it may well be necessary to raise the concentration (dose) of antagonist to maintain a given degree of β-blockade.

Turning to the specific cardiac actions of noradrenaline, there are four main effects which are paralleled by direct sympathetic stimulation of the heart.

1) an increase in the frequency of the heart beat
2) an increase in the rate of tension development and in the peak tension developed in the myocardium (often loosely called an increase in "contractility")
3) an increase in conduction velocity of electrical impulses through atria, atrio-ventricular node, the Purkinje system and ventricles
4) there is an increased tendency of Purkinje fibres to exhibit pacemaker activity and an increased risk of ventricular fibrillation.

All these effects are mediated through β-adrenoceptors and are sensitive to inhibition by β-adrenoceptor antagonists.

CARDIAC ARRHYTHMIAS

If we compare the electrical action potential of cells in the SA node with atrial muscle fibres we see a clear difference. Whereas the muscle fibre potential has a stable resting voltage, that of the pacemaker cell exhibits a gradual rise preceeding the rapid depolarization. This is variously termed pacemaker prepotential, spontaneous depolarization or diastolic depolarization. Similar properties have been observed from transmembrane potential recordings in the atrio-ventricular node, the bundle of His and the Purkinje system. It is the electrophysiological basis of cardiac automaticity. The SA node is normally dominant by virtue of the highest frequency of signal generation. The slope of diastolic depolarization is sensitive to both noradrenaline and acetylcholine. The observed effect of noradrenaline is to accelerate the rate of depolarization of the pre-potential. This means that the slope of diastolic depolarization is increased, the membrane potential falls more rapidly and the rate of spontaneous discharge increases. Conversely acetylcholine, or vagal stimulation, decreases the slope of the prepotentials is decreased and the rate of firing slows down (Fig. 3). The shortening or lengthening of the time interval between attainment of maximal depolarization and reaching threshold voltage to enter phase O of the cardiac action potential is the electrophysiological basis of sinus tachycardia and sinus bradycardia respectively (Hutter and Trautwein, 1956). The electrochemical basis of this phenomenon is less secure. It was earlier thought that the effect of noradrenaline was due to an increase in the rate at which potassium permeability declines between action potentials or to an increase in the

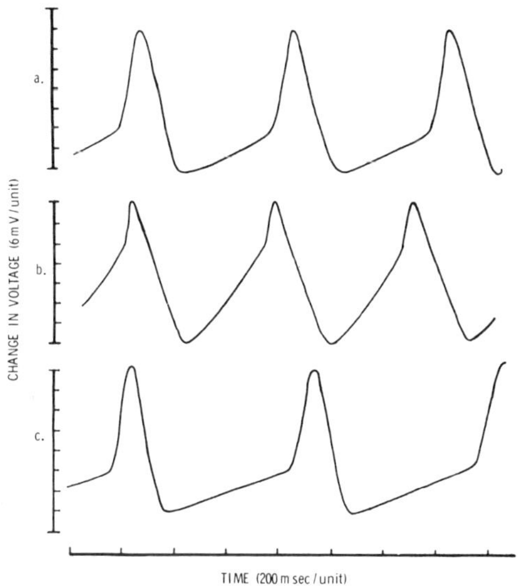

Figure 3.

Action potentials from single pacemaker cells in rabbit atria in vitro; (a) control study; (b) 45 sec. after local application of 1-adrenaline; (c) 40 sec. after application of acetylcholine. Note particularly the change in slope of prepotential and rate of firing. (after West, Falk and Cervoni, 1956. J. Pharmac. exp. Ther., 117, 245.)

number of sodium channels carrying the rapid inward sodium current. It now seems more likely that there is a noradrenaline-induced increase in the slow inward positive calcium current responsible for the acceleration of diastolic depolarization.

Much work has been published relating the positive inotropic actions of noradrenaline to an intracellular accumulation of cyclic-AMP following activation of adenylate cyclase. Until recently, however, there was little evidence to link changes in the concentration of the cyclic nucleotide with changes in cardiac rate. In elegant experiments Tsien (1973) has now demonstrated acceleration of diastolic depolarization in cardiac muscle following intracellular application of cyclic-AMP by iontophoresis through micropipettes.

Inherent rhythmicity is a property of all parts of the myocardium and conduction system. Under abnormal conditions any part can become the cardiac pacemaker. For example this can happen when the SA node is depressed, when the bundle of His is interrupted or when an abnormal or ectopic focus in atria or ventricles discharges faster than the SA node.

Four types of cardiac dysrhythmia are particularly sensitive to β-adrenoceptor antagonists:

1) catecholamine-induced e.g. under anaesthesia
2) atrial flutter/fibrillation
3) paroxysmal atrial tachycardia
4) digitalis-induced arrhythmias.

In all cases it is possible to trace a logical role for these drugs by virtue of their selective anti-sympathetic activity. Reduction in noradrenaline stimulated frequency or facilitation of conduction through the A-V node account for categories 1 to 3 whether due to an increase in circulating catecholamine levels, excess sympathetic discharge or an imbalance between the autonomic control mechanism. There is, however, uncertainty about the mechanism involved in the correction of digitalis arrhythmias. My personal belief is that the confusion stems from uncritical extrapolation of experimental results from laboratory to clinic. First it must be agreed that many β-adrenoceptor antagonists also possess the less specific property of membrane stabilization. By this is meant the ability to decrease the permeability of neuronal or muscle membranes to the rapid influx of sodium and potassium ions associated with impulse conduction. This may be reflected in the inhibition of passage of propagated action potentials in motor nerves, local anaesthesia or a decrease in the maximum rate of rise of an atrial action potential. This latter property has been linked with the antiarrhythmic activity of quinidine giving rise to use of the term "quinidine-like" to describe the actions of some β-blocking drugs. In all cases the concentrations of β-adrenoceptor antagonist required to demonstrate such membrane stabilising effects are substantially greater than those required to cancel sympathetic stimulation. In 1966, Howe and Shanks reported that both isomers of propranolol were equally effective in reversing established digitalis-induced arrhythmias in dogs. As β-adrenoceptor antagonists the (−)-isomer was many times more effective than the

(+)-isomer. Many other investigators have confirmed these observations and extended them to other compounds in the β-blocking category. Hence the belief that the correction of digitalis toxicity depended on some property other than β-adrenoceptor blockade. Yet from these studies in dogs where doses of up to 5 mg/kg, intravenously, of propranolol were required to achieve the effect the clinical implications were ignored. They are that doses of up to 35p mg, in a single bolus injection might be required intravenously to correct a bigeminal rhythm or ventricular tachycardia associated with digitalis toxicity. Few clinicians would care to experiment on this scale and where clinical benefit from propranolol is observed in this context, a dose of 10 mg repeated once or twice is only rarely exceeded.

One little known piece of pharmacology is that depletion of catecholamines from tissue stores in experimental animals by reserpine-like drugs, greatly increases the resistance to the toxicity of cardiac glycosides (Ciofalo, Levitt and Roberts, 1967). In some way, therefore, it is highly probable that the experimental toxicity seen in laboratory models is a complex interplay between sympathetic and digitalis activity. It would not be surprising if the removal of the sympathetic component by β-blockade should alter the sensitivity to the proarrhythmic potential of cardiac glycosides.

An alternative approach to experiments in which reversion of an established arrhythmia is attempted has been a favourite of Dr. Vaughan Williams (1970 for review). In his experiments animals (usually guinea-pigs) are pretreated with the prospective antiarrhythmic agent. The threshold for the appearance of various indices of arrhythmic activity is then determined. For convenience I have extracted a number of results from Dr. Vaughan William's recent papers with a view to consolidating my argument that β-adrenoceptor blockade is of paramount importance rather than any other pharmacological property.

The comparative protective action of the isomers of propranolol with that of practolol is illustrated in Fig. 4. The isomers of propranolol are approximately equi-active in depressing phase O of the cardiac action potential and practolol is at least 100 times less active than either. The antiarrhythmic activity of practolol, however, parallels that of (-)-propranolol. Further the potency ratio between these curves is identical with that for conventional β blocking activity in a number of species i.e. practolol is 40% or $2\frac{1}{2}$ times less active than propranolol.

A further comparison between the anti-fibrillatory effects of three adrenoceptor antagonists which differ in potency both as β-blockers and as local anaesthetics is also instructive (Fig. 5). Pindolol is more active than propranolol which is more active than INPEA against isoprenaline-induced tachycardia. Propranolol is more active than pindolol in depressing cardiac action potentials whilst INPEA is without effect in

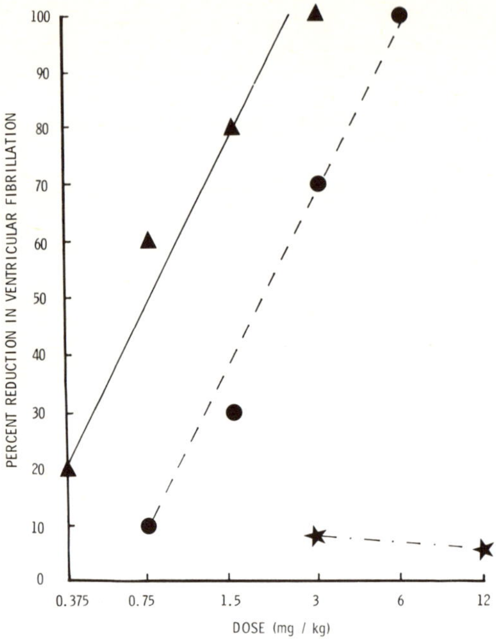

Figure 4.

A comparison of the anti-fibrillatory effects of (-)-propranolol (▲——▲), practolol (●——●) and (+)-propranolol (*——*) in guinea-pigs when ouabain was used as the pro-arrhythmic agent. (After Dohadwalla, Freedberg and Vaughan Williams, 1969, Br. J. Pharmac., 36, 257; and Papp and Vaughan Williams, 1969, ibid, 37, 391).

this context. The anti-fibrillatory action again parallels β-blocking potency.

One of the most convincing pieces of evidence comes from the studies

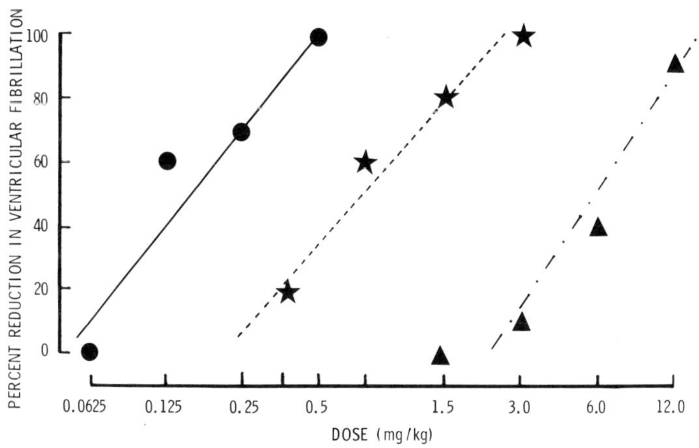

Figure 5.

A comparison of the anti-fibrillatory effects of pindolol (●———●), (-)-propranolol (*———*) and INPEA (▲———▲) in guinea-pigs when ouabain was used as the pro-arrhythmic agent. (After Dohadwalla, Freedberg and Vaughan Williams, 1969, Br. J. Pharmac., 36, 257; and Singh and Vaughan Williams, 1971, ibid, 43, 10.).

of Dr. Gibson (personal communication). He has compared the effects of propranolol on ventricular ectopic beats and exercise tachycardia. For any given blood level of propranolol the inhibition of either exercise tachycardia or ectopic beats was similar, the effect/concentration curves being virtually superimposable.

It seems certain that the β-adrenoceptor antagonist action itself is responsible for all types of antiarrhythmic activity observed in this group of drugs. The problem of concurrent depression of cardiac contractility is also most probably a consequence of removal of sympathetic support and not due to any direct action on muscle contraction. Not all β-blocking drugs, especially practolol, produce a decrease in cardiac output when used in dysrhythmic situations. Whether this is a consequence of partial agonist activity or a reduced peripheral component on venous return remains to be established.

ANGINA PECTORIS

Angina pectoris is a sympatomatic of progressive vascular degeneration within the myocardium. The acute pain is related to a sudden imbalance between the oxygen supply and the oxygen demand. Deposition of lipid with narrowing and decreasing elasticity of coronary arterial vessels compromises the flexibility of coronary blood flow so characteristic of the healthy heart. The appearance of anginal pain is indicative that the oxygen supply cannot meet the requirements of a given cardiac performance. There are only two therapeutic options. Either the supply of blood and oxygen must be increased or the work of the heart must be limited. Improvements in coronary blood flow are not a pract ical proposition in the clinical situation except by surgical means. Limitation of cardiac work may be achieved either by decreasing the external after-load, or peripheral resistance, or by decreasing cardiac work directly.

The organic nitrates, long miscalled coronary vasodilators, are now believed to exert their undoubted beneficial actions by reduction of arterial resistance in the peripheral circulation thus decreasing the pressure against which the heart must expel its systolic volume. The alternative therapy is to use specific antagonists of sympathetic stimulation of the heart - the β-adrenoceptor antagonists.

It is appropriate to review those factors which govern myocardial oxygen consumption. There are four principal factors:

1) heart rate

2) left ventricular systolic pressure

3) rate of tension development in left ventricular muscle

4) heart size.

Additionally there may be alterations in myocardial oxygen consumption as a direct consequence of changes in metabolic substrate availability e.g. glucose and free fatty acids.

Stimulation of the heart by sympathetic nerve fibres will result in an increase in heart rate, systolic ejection pressure and dP/dT but will bring about a reduction in heart size. There is much evidence to suggest that such changes are a consistent feature of the response to exercise and other precipitating causes of angina such as exposure to cold or emotional disturbance (Robinson, 1971).

Specific antagonism of the cardiac sympathetic response would result in reduced increase in heart rate, reduced rate of development of tension in ventricular muscle and reduced systolic ejection pressure. These three effects would spare myocardial oxygen consumption. On the other hand, sympathetic blockade will lead to an increase in resting diastolic fibre length and an overall increase in heart size (Chamberlain, 1966a). This leads to an increased requirement for oxygen supply. Clinical benefit from specific blockade of the cardiac sympathetic response will depend therefore on the balance of these four effects.

Extensive clinical trials of β-adrenoceptor antagonists in angina pectoris now produce indisputable evidence of a beneficial action. It would appear therefore that the reduction in heart rate, tension development and left ventricular systolic pressure outweigh the disadvantage of ventricular enlargement in the majority of patients. Most investigators now seem to favour the view that it is the reduction in heart rate both at rest and during exercise which is the most important effect (see Taylor, 1973).

Much has been written concerning the so-called "oxygen wasting effect" of catecholamines, the transmitter substances which transfer electrical impulses from sympathetic nerve fibres to the heart muscle. In addition to the haemodynamic effects of sympathetic stimulation outlined above, there are also metabolic effects principally an increase in lipolysis and glycogenolysis. The consequence of lipolysis is an increase

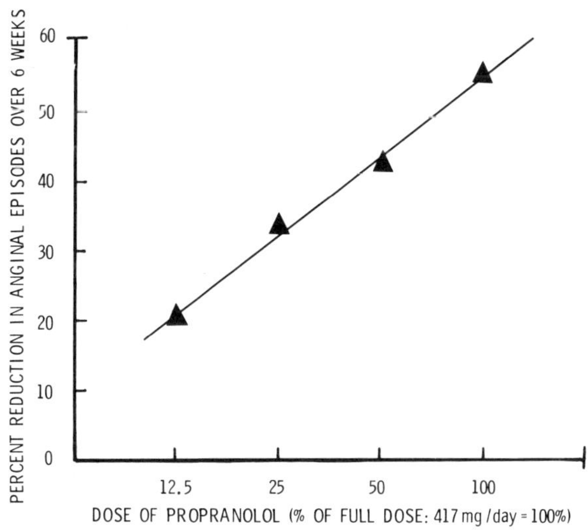

Figure 6.

Relationship between dose of propranolol and relative effect on frequency of anginal episodes (n = 16). Each patient was titrated to dose yielding maximum benefit and then given 12.5, 25, 50 or 100% of that dose for 6 week periods. No. of episodes in 6 week placebo period was 85 ± 26 (After Prochard and Gillam, 1971; Br. Heart J., 33, 473.

in the circulating levels of free fatty acids. From studies of isolated perfused hearts it was concluded that high concentrations of fatty acids increased myocardial oxygen consumption (Challoner and Steinberg, 1966a, b). One way of imitating these experiments *in vivo* is to infuse a fat emulsion with heparin in dogs. The heparin will activate plasma lipoprotein lipase and accelerate breakdown of the fat and so rapidly raise free fatty acid levels. In such experiments free fatty acid levels rose approximately six-fold, from 500 to 3000 μEq/litre but without change in haemodynamic variables. The measured myocardial oxygen consumption rose however from 8.6 to 10.7 ml/min per 100 g of muscle, an increase of 26% which was statistically very highly significant (Mjøs, 1971a). Such changes in FFA are also observed after sympathetic stimulation and can be mimicked by the intravenous infusion of isoprenaline. In this case, however, there will also be a change in haemodynamic measurements. In these experiments, the FFA level rose from 500 to 1000 μEq/l, but heart rate by 25 beats per minute and both dP/dT and cardiac output doubled. The myocardial oxygen consumption rose from 9.9 to 17.6 ml/min per 100 g. It is possible to prevent the rise in FFA selectively by using nicotinic acid, without altering the haemodynamic responses to isoprenaline (Mjøs, 1971b). Under these conditions, when the FFA response was completely inhibited the myocardial oxygen consumption rose from 9.7 to 14.2 ml/min per 100 g yet the rise in heart rate and dP/dT was unchanged. By preventing the associated lipolysis from sympathetic stimulation, myocardial oxygen consumption rose by only 46% by comparison with 78% increase under control conditions when FFA levels had doubled (Mjos, 1971b). This represents a reduction of 32% in myocardial oxygen consumption for an equivalent amount of cardiac work under isoprenaline stimulation when FFA mobilization is prevented.

Studies in man show that stress situations such as centrifugation, racing car driving or rock-climbing all produce significant elevations of plasma free fatty acid levels (Glaister, Harrison and Allnutt, 1973; Taggart and Carruthers, 1971). These responses can be blocked by administration of β-adrenoceptor antagonists since the receptor mechanism governing cardiac sympathetic responses appears to be very similar to that governing lipolysis (Taggart and Carruthers, 1972). It is highly probable, therefore, that in anginal patients additional benefit, in terms of reduced myocardial oxygen demand, comes from suppression of lipolysis.

With the exception of sotalol and propranolol, all the other β-adrenoceptor antagonists possess some capacity to stimulate cardiac function (Barrett and Carter, 1970). Interestingly this seems to be predominantly a rate effect rather than an inotropic action. Such activity can be detected in animals depleted of endogenous catecholamines. The question of importance is whether or not this property constitutes any clinical advantage. Barrett and Nunn (1971) performed experiments using a guinea-pig heart lung preparation. Under control conditions survival with constant cardiac output was obtained for about 6 hr. Addition of pentobarbitone, however, brought about premature failure. If the β-adrenoceptor stimulant isoprenaline was also added then survival could be prolonged by up to 100%. At the point when the preparations would have died in the absence of isoprenaline, two β-adrenoceptor antagonists were administered separately, propranolol having the least and dichloroisoprenaline having the greatest partial agonist or intrinsic sympathomimetic activity. Doses were selected which had no deleterious action on the preparation *per se* and which were pharmacologically equivalent in β-blocking potency. Both agents produced a rapid failure of the preparations. It was concluded that in a life-threatening situation the partial agonist properties do not confer any significant benefit in terms of safety.

It was recognized early on that the use of β-adrenoceptor antagonists in patients with asthma could provoke bronchoconstriction. A search was made therefore for compounds which might exert a selective action on cardiac function whilst sparing β-adrenoceptors in the bronchial tree. From these studies, it was found that practolol differed from propranolol in that for a given degree of cardiac antagonism to the responses to isoprenaline there was a failure to prevent the vasodilatation. The degree of separation between cardiac effects of propranolol and practolol, was about three whereas the degree of separation in the vasodepressor response was nearer 400. Experiments in guinea-pigs, protected from the fatal bronchoconstrictor action of histamine by isoprenaline, showed a similar differentiation of effect between the two drugs. In this case practolol was 150 times less active than propranolol. It is important to recognise that this difference between the two drugs is relative and not absolute. It was for this reason that I coined the term "cardio-selective" in relation to practolol. Although there is an implied margin of safety there is no guarantee that practolol will not induce bronchospasm in susceptible individuals.

Subsequent studies revealed two important differences between propranolol and practolol not yet mentioned. Firstly their metabolism by animals and man is quite distinct. Whereas propranolol is extensively metabolised and has a short half-life of about 2 hr, practolol is 85% excreted unchanged and has a half-life of 10-12 hr (Fitzgerald and Scales, 1968). This is the scientific basis for the recommendation of 6 hourly, or 4 times a day dosing with propranolol, compared with 12 hourly i.e. twice daily for practolol. Taking into account their difference in potency, a patient responding to propranolol 40 mg four times daily might be expected to require practolol 200 mg twice daily.

The second major difference is the failure of practolol to provide adequate and comparable antagonism to the positive chronotropic actions of isoprenaline in conscious animals and man (Brick, Hutchinson, McDevitt, Roddie and Shanks, 1968). This represents a difference in response in conscious dogs and anaesthetized animals where effective dose-related inhibition of isoprenaline-induced tachycardia is demonstrable (Barrett, 1969). In man, there is a similar disparity between the efficacy of a newer cardio-selective β-adrenoceptor antagonist, I.C.I. 66082, and propranolol where both agents are comparable in their ability to suppress exercise-induced tachycardia but only propranolol has a significant inhibitory effect on isoprenaline-induced tachycardia, at the same dose levels (McGibney, 1974). From experiments in dogs, it has been argued that the apparent failure of cardio-selective antagonists to attenuate the tachycardia due to isoprenaline, stems from vagal inhibition consequent upon the unopposed concomitant hypotensive effect of isoprenaline (Barrett, 1971). Recent studies clearly indicate that variation in vagal influence can alter heart rate positively or negatively following section of the sympathetic nerves to the heart (Norman and Whitwam, 1974). A comparative study of practolol versus isoprenaline-induced tachycardia is conscious and anaesthetized man is not yet available. The implication of these results is that the conventional use of isoprenaline which combines both positive chronotropic and vasodilator actions is not appropriate in the assessment of cardio-selective β-adrenoceptor antagonists. Other methods including exercise and glyceryl trinitrate administration are currently under evaluation.

The question of the contribution of β-blocking properties and membrane stabilizing activity in the relief of anginal pain has been answered from clinical experiments. Measurement of effort tolerance in anginal subjects on a bicycle ergometer showed a significant prolongation of exercise time to pain for both propranolol and practolol. Administration of an equivalent weight of (+)-propranolol (which has equal membrane stabilizing activity but only one fiftieth the β-blocking activity of propranolol (Barrett and Cullum, 1968)), had no effect on effort tolerance (Wilson, Brooke, Lloyd and Robinson, 1969). There is other evidence which confirms that the β-blocking activity of this class of drugs is necessary for anti-anginal action rather than the ancillary pharmacological properties. For example partial agonist or intrinsic sympathomimetic activity appears to be equally unimportant as the membrane stabilizing property. Oxprenolol and propranolol have a similar anti-anginal activity (Thadani, Sharma, Meeran, Majid, Whitaker and Taylor, 1974) yet only the former displays partial agonist actions (Barrett and Carter, 1970). Furthermore practolol, which lacks membrane stabilizing properties, is a partial agonist and is cardio-selective has similar anti-anginal activity to oxprenolol and propranolol both of which block all β-adrenoceptors indiscriminately at dose levels producing a similar reduction in exercise heart rate (Prichard, Aellig and Richardson, 1970). The contribution of central sedative action is probably insignificant from the fact that propranolol readily enters the brain whereas practolol does not pass the blood brain barrier (Scales and Cosgrove, 1970). Both these drugs possess similar anti-anginal activity at dose levels adjusted to produce equivalent reduction in exercising heart rate (Coltart, 1971). To quote Taylor (1973), "these arguments lend strong support to the view that the ancillary properties so far described for the different β-adrenoceptor antagonists are of little theoretical relevance or practical importance in the treatment of angina pectoris."

HYPERTENSION

The use of β-adrenoceptor antagonists in the management of hypertension derives from clinical observations. During their laboratory development, an exploitable hypotensive action was not foreseen. As long ago as 1964, Prichard prospectively evaluated pronethalol in a group of eleven hypertensives over a 3 month period. There was a mean fall in supine pressure of 33/23 mm Hg and no evidence of postural hypotension. This followed an earlier observation when a 14 day treatment with pronethalol in anginal subjects produced a modest fall in blood pressure (Prichard et al., 1963). Prichard (1964) claimed that intravenous pronethalol did not lower blood pressure acutely in man whereas Black and Stephenson (1962) had found that it did so in anaesthetized cats. Prichard infused 100 mg (1.4 mg/kg) over 10 minutes whereas Black and Stephenson (1962) gave 5 mg/kg in a bolus injection. The different conditions do not permit the frequent statement that β-blockers lower blood pressure acutely in animals but not in man. From the evidence available it would be fairer to conclude that intravenous administration of β-adrenoceptor antagonists is not associated with a lowering of blood pressure at dose levels adequate to reduce heart rate.

Over the last 10 years many reports have been published in which a significant lowering of blood pressure has been achieved by use of β-adrenoceptor antagonists. These include propranolol (Prichard and Gillam, 1966), oxprenolol (Dorph and Binder, 1969), alprenolol (Furberg and Michaelson, 1969), practolol (Leishman et al., 1970) and pindolol (Morgan et al., 1972). Between them these drugs share a variety of additional properties including membrane stabilizing actions, partial agonist (intrinsic sympathomimetic) activity and cardioselectivity. They also vary in potency as β-adrenoceptor antagonists e.g. pindolol > propranolol > practolol. The same order of potency can be seen in the clinical anti-hypertensive studies of Zacharias et al. (1973) and Stokes et al. (1974). Further, in a case taken from Prichard (1971) in which (+)-propranolol was substituted for (±)-propranolol following stabilization of hypotensive response to the racemic compound, there was a sudden increase in both mean pressure and heart rate. After one week (±)-propranolol was instituted again at the same dose level (100 mg q.d.s.) with prompt recontrol of the blood pressure (Fig. 7). Taken together these arguments begin to suggest that β-adrenoceptor antagonism is the

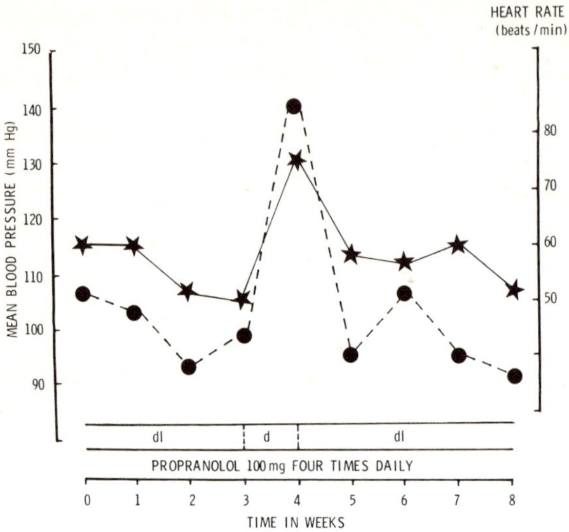

Figure 7.

Mean blood pressure (• ——— •) and heart rate (*——— *) in an individual patient with hypertension controlled by dl-propranolol, 100 mg q.d.s. At week 3 an equal amount of d-propranolol was substituted, for 7 days, followed by re-institution of dl-propranolol (After Prichard, 1971).

common property leading to a reduction in blood pressure. From time to time one hears anecdotes that anti-hypertensive therapy with β-adrenoceptor antagonists derives from a central depressant action producing a "zombie-like" state. But there are also stories of a-methyl dopa producing such decreased mental agility that jobs have been lost only to be regained when transferred to a β-adrenoceptor antagonist, with equivalent control of blood pressure. Without supporting evidence such stories should be disregarded since they only do harm and may prejudice positive clinical management.

In relation to the maintenance of blood pressure β-adrenoceptor antagonists may be expected to affect cardiac function rather than peripheral resistance. Sympathetic control of arteriolar calibre is mediated via α-adrenoceptors for which there are other specific antagonists e.g. phenoxybenzamine, phentolamine, thymoxamine. Effective β-adrenoceptor blockade would not be associated with any inhibition of the splanchnic vasoconstrictor response to postural change. In contrast, inhibition of β-adrenoceptors at vasodilator sites will serve to enhance the pressor response to adrenaline. This is of importance in phaeochromocytoma but is not considered of general physiological significance without acute pharmacological experiments.

Possible Mechanisms and Hypotensive Action

It is true that from the days of hexamethonium onwards (i.e. 1951) many attempts to develop anti-hypertensive medicines have taken an impirical view. Elevated pressure may be lowered by decreasing peripheral resistance, cardiac output, blood volume or blood viscosity. Sympatholytic activity, in the broadest sense, to reduce peripheral resistance has been the commonest aim. Ganglionic blockade, depletion of transmitter, prevention of release of transmitter, facilitation of enzymic degradation, substitution of false transmitter substrate, a-adrenoceptor antagonists and central vasomotor depression are all represented in todays list of available hypotensive agents. It is interesting to note, however, that the more effective agents include a cardiac as well as a peripheral component in their mode of action. For example, guanethidine which is actively taken up by adrenergic neurones and then prevents further transmitter release, is as active in myocardial sites as in arteriolar muscle sites.

The β-adrenoceptor antagonists exert powerful effects on cardiac function and it was natural to see an explanation of hypotensive actions on this basis. As we shall see this was not wholly profitable.

Before going on to consider the possible mechanisms of action it may be helpful to consider both dosage and onset of action. In most cases the degree of β-adrenoceptor blockade is assessed acutely in response to a specific stimulus e.g. isoprenaline (Ulrych et al., 1968) or amyl nitrite (Franciosa et al., 1973). Such a test is indicative of an acute degree of block but does not forecast the requirement for 24 hr a day, 7 days per week inhibition. Chamberlain (1966b) showed that 50 mg of propranolol produced an effect 75% that of thoracic sympathectomy in man for about 2 hr. From this we might predict a total daily dose of the order of 600 mg per day in angina or hypertension. Further many trials are designed to show a significant difference between drug and placebo. Selected dose levels may not be the same as those necessary for maximal clinical response. Finally, in outpatient studies it may be necessary for patients to attend for several consecutive visits until an appropriate dose level is reached. Care must be taken not to confuse this situation with a delayed onset of action. Before citing studies it is advisable to study the small print in the methods section with some care.

Involvement of Baroreceptors

In their earlier report, Prichard and Gillam (1966) reported an impression that the full hypotensive effect of propranolol took some weeks to reach its maximum. Subsequently (Prichard and Gillam, 1969), they followed a number of patients and their response to propranolol over 3 months. Although there was no significant difference in the hypotensive response at 1 month and 3 months, it appeared that the decrease in heart rate was immediate whilst pressure fell gradually over the first three weeks. The study is defective in that daily pressure measurements were not made over the critical period. From this apparent temporal dissociation of cardiac and pressure effects, Prichard and Gillam proposed that the baroreceptors were gradually conditioned by reduced pressor responses to regulate the blood pressure at a lower level. It was envisaged that β-adrenoceptor blockade would protect the heart against the cardiac sympathetic component to various stimuli known to activate the baroreceptor reflex. This has been disputed (Tarazi and Dustan, 1972). Other workers, notably Lydtin et al., (1972) and Buhler et al. (1972) have noted falls in blood pressure within 48 hr. Franciosa et al. (1973) also claimed a definite reduction in blood pressure with the analogue, timolol, but that the effect became more pronounced with continuation of therapy. Unfortunately, close inspection of their data suggests that anticipation of treatment was more effective than medication itself although the rebound on withdrawal was more impressive. It is regrettable that workers do not read each others papers more carefully before citing them since Franciosa et al. (1973) comment that their results differ from those of Prichard and Gillam (1969); careful inspection of the published data shows no true comparison of data to be possible. At the present time it is not possible to adduce any evidence in support of the baroreceptor hypothesis and indeed difficult to envisage any means of assessing such a phenomenon in man.

Involvement of Metabolites

Oral administration of propranolol results in significant metabolism to the 4-hydroxy analogue, a compound having equivalent β-adrenoceptor antagonist activity but with a considerably longer half life (Paterson et al., 1970). It has been suggested that this may be the effective agent in controlling blood pressure during propranolol medication (Hansson et al.,

1971). There is no evidence for this suggestion but even if it were true it still fails to afford any insight into the mechanism of the hypotensive effect. Additional metabolites of propranolol arise from removal of the N-isopropyl group of the side chain yielding α-naphthoxylactic acid and isopropylamine (Hayes and Cooper, 1971; Tindell, Walle and Gaffney, 1972). Pharmacological analysis of the effects of isopropylamine showed it to have effects on the cardiovascular system which might involve decreased sympathetic transmission (Walle, Ishizaki and Gaffney, 1972). Subsequent studies have suggested, however, that amounts produced in therapeutic situations are probably too small to have any cardiovascular significance (Bakke, Davies, Davies and Dollery, 1973). Although the balance of evidence does not favour an anti-hypertensive action as the result of direct or cumulative effects of relatively simple metabolites it remains a possibility.

Involvement of Central Nervous System

A number of investigators have proposed a central nervous system effect of β-adrenoceptor antagonists in the reported hypotensive actions. Impetus for such hypotheses stems from two sources:

a) the rapid penetration of propranolol into the brain (Masouka and Hansson, 1967)

b) c.n.s. depressant activities of propranolol sufficient to classify it as a sedative and anti-convulsant (Leszkovszky and Tardos,

1965; Murman et al., 1966; Bainbridge and Greenwood, 1971).

Experiments in anaesthetized cats (Kelliher and Buckley, 1970) claimed to show that intraventricular administration of either (±)- or (+)-propranolol lowered systemic blood pressure significantly. But the amounts of drug employed were 0.5 mg per 0.1 ml of artificial C.S.F. - a concentration of 5 mg/ml. Propranolol in both racemic and isomeric forms, is a powerful membrane stabilising agent and such concentrations are more than adequate to completely block conduction in sheathed amphibian motor nerves (Barrett and Cullum, 1968). More recently, Dollery et al. (1973) have studied the effects of propranolol following intracerebroventricular administration in conscious rabbits. Injection of 500 μg (±)-propranolol produced a prompt rise in mean blood pressure which was followed by a prolonged fall (Fig. 8). Equal amounts of (+)-propranolol or procaine (1 mg) also elicited the prompt elevation of pressure but no late fall. It appears that the minimum effective dose is 100 μg for (-)-propranolol but that no activity from practolol has been observed (Lewis, personal communication). Experiments of a similar nature in conscious cats also showed a fall in blood pressure following the injection of propranolol 500-600 μg into lateral cerebral ventricles and additionally bradycardia, but no initial pressor response (Day and Roach, 1973). In these studies isoprenaline (15-60 μg) by the same route produced an increase in blood pressure and heart rate, augmented

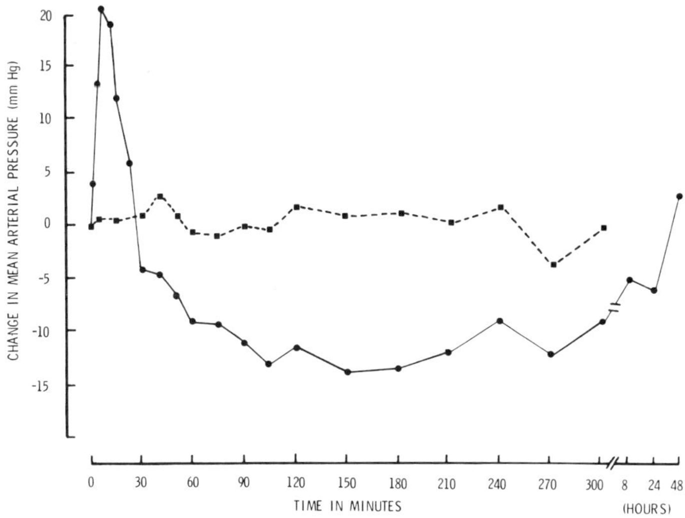

Figure 8.

Changes in mean arterial pressure in conscious rabbits after 500 μg of l-propranolol intra-cerebroventricularly (●——●) (n = 9) and intravenously (■——■) (n = 7). (After Reid, Lewis, Myers and Dollery, 1974).

by cholinergic blockade but antagonized by i.c.v. pretreatment with propranolol. Such results were not confirmed in conscious dogs where i.c.v. propranolol (600 μg) did not alter heart rate or blood pressure (Conway and Lang, 1974). In these experiments there was no hypertensive response from isoprenaline (50 μg i.c.v.) although higher doses raised heart rate and lowered pressure. The isoprenaline responses in dogs were abolished by i.c.v. propranolol (600 μg or 2 mg) but these doses were also effective in preventing tachycardia and the vasodepressor response to intravenous isoprenaline (1-2 μg/kg). Although these findings are of interest, particularly the (-)-isomer of propranolol dependent delayed hypotensive response (Dollery et al., 1973), they do not represent conclusive evidence of a central component in the human responsiveness to β-adrenoceptor antagonists.

Central nervous system side-effects of β-adrenoceptor antagonists have been widely reported (Prichard and Gillam, 1969; Simpson and Waal-Manning, 1970; Morgan et al., 1972) when these drugs are used in anti-hypertensive therapy which might infer a central component to the observed clinical response. In the experiments of Dusting and Rand (1974) propranolol was shown to lower pressure in DOCA/salt-treated hypertensive rats at dose levels which did not block cardiac β-adrenoceptors (0.2 mg/kg subcutaneously). As in many other studies an action on the central nervous system is implicated but not proven. Perhaps the greatest difficulty in accepting a central mechanism of action is that cardiovascular reflexes are not obviously impaired following clinical use of β-adrenoceptor antagonists to lower blood pressure. A mechanism lowering peripheral resistance without affecting the response to change in posture must be envisaged but as yet there is no direct evidence to support such a notion and there is much against it.

Adjustments to Decreased Cardiac Output

The most attractive hypotheses center on the long-term adjustment to a chronic reduction in cardiac output. From the earliest measurements of the haemodynamic consequences of β-adrenoceptor blockade a reduction in cardiac output has been a consistent acute finding. In subjects with labile hypertension an elevated cardiac output is common and it was logical to attribute the hypotensive action of propranolol to this cause (Frohlich et al., 1968). Although reduction in cardiac output occurs soon after the drug is given there was no fall in blood pressure in normotensive or hypertensive individuals. Whilst the degree of bradycardia was significantly greater in hypertensive subjects, it indicates that the elevated blood pressure was not maintained by the elevated cardiac output (Ulrych et al., 1968). In a long term study of propranolol in 52 subjects, Tarazi and Dustan (1972) made repeated haemodynamic studies. They concluded that the initial haemodynamic values could not be used to predict responsiveness. Just over half the patients were classified as "non-responders". In those who did respond there was no difference between those with essential or renovascular hypertension. Cardiac output was reduced in both groups i.e. with or without a hypotensive response which suggested a change in peripheral resistance of those who did respond. Tarazi and Dustan (1972) suggest that patients responding to propranolol may experience some change in autoregulation but in plain words they are baffled and cannot adduce a consistent haemodynamic explanation of the observed effects. Further confirmation of the inadequacy of a haemodynamic mechanism comes from the timolol study (Franciosa et al., 1973) where in a comparison with propranolol equivalent hypotensive effects were apparent after 5 weeks but whereas cardiac output was reduced by 23% in the propranolol group it was marginally higher in the timolol group. In this study peripheral resistance was slightly lower in the timolol group but clearly increased in the propranolol-treated patients.

Adrenergic Neurone Blockade

From time to time reports have appeared in which evidence of adrenergic neurone blocking activity has been suggested for some β-adrenoceptor antagonists (Day et al., 1968; Ganguly and Bhattacharya, 1970; Mylecharane and Raper, 1970; 1973; Barrett and Nunn, 1970; Eliash and Weinstock, 1971). Although some of the evidence in preparations such as guinea-pig vas deferens, rabbit ear artery and cat nictitating membrane is pharmacologically sound, it is difficult to distinguish between such a specific property as adrenergic neurone blockade and the less specific consequences of membrane stabilizing action. It appears that characteristic guanethidien-like properties can be demonstrated at concentrations of propranolol at 200 ng/ml (Mylecharane and Raper, 1973) whereas at 20 μg/ml, the inhibition of sympathetic conduction is due to membrane stabilization. The blood levels of propranolol associated with a maximal blockade of exertional tachycardia in man were approximately 100 ng/ml (Coltart and Shand, 1970) which implies that clinical adrenergic neurone blockade from propranolol is a possibility. Practical arguments against this explanation for anti-hypertensive action come from studies in which thoraco-lumbar sympathetic stimulation was employed as a vasoconstrictor stimulus. Neither in anaesthetized dogs (Dawes and Faulkner, 1974) nor pithed rats (Dusting and Rand, 1974) did propranolol exert a significant inhibitory action on the induced pressor response whereas guanethidine did do so. Perhaps more importantly, in man, no evidence of orthostatic hypotension or failure of ejaculation have been reported during the treatment of hypertension with β-adrenoceptor antagonists.

An interesting pharmacological question is raised by the observation that the adrenergic neuron blocking properties of propranolol, at lower concentrations, are shared by its own (+)-isomer and by sotalol and its optical isomers (Mylecharane and Raper, 1973). Presumably it is necessary for any potential adrenergic neuron blocking agent to be taken up selectively in the adrenergic neuron. In the case of propranolol this may well occur by diffusional exchange by virtue of its lipophilicity. But the polar nature of sotalol implies that uptake would require an active process yet its N-isopropyl substitution would surely prevent it being a substrate for the $Uptake_1$ pathway (Burgen and Iversen, 1965).

Involvement of renin Secretion

The most exciting development in the search for an explanation of the hypotensive actions of β-adrenoceptor antagonists is related to renin secretion. The relationship between biogenic amines, sympathetic nerves and renin secretion have been reviewed by Ganong (1973). To quote from his abstract "the secretion of renin is increased by sympathetic stimulation. Renin secretion is affected by arteriolar baroreceptor and a mechanism which operates through the macula densa, but the bulk of the evidence indicates that the sympathetic effects are independent of these controlling influences. Instead the sympathetic effects are mediated via β-adrenoceptors and there is reason to believe that the receptors involved are located on the cell membranes of the juxtoglomerular cells themselves. The juxtoglomerular cells respond to circulating catecholamines and to catecholamines released by the adrenergic neurones in the renal arterioles." The increase in renin secretion produced by hypoglycaemia (Assaykeen et al., 1970), electrical stimulation of the pressor region of the medulla oblongata (Passo et al., 1971), renal nerve stimulation (Loeffler et al., 1972) or infusion of catecholamines (Assaykeen and Ganong, 1971) is inhibited by propranolol but unaffected by phenoxybenzamine. The specific β-adrenoceptor nature of the response is confirmed in man where the elevation of plasma renin activity on standing was dramatically reduced by (±)-propranolol but unaffected by (+)-propranolol (Tolbert et al., 1973). Involvement of cyclic AMP is suggested by the observation that theophylline stimulates renin secretion but that this is unaffected by either α- or β-adrenoceptor antagonists (Reid et al., 1972).

Inhibition of renin secretion by propranolol (Buhler et al., 1972) and alprenolol (Castenfors et al., 1973) has been reported in man. This may not be a general property of all β-adrenoceptor antagonists since pindolol (LB 46) apparently stimulates renin secretion in rabbits (Weber et al., 1972). The fact that pindolol is a potent partial agonist (Barrett and Carter, 1970) may be a complicating factor since isoprenaline itself also raises renin secretion rates. Practolol has also been shown to reduce the renin response to tilting in patients in whom it was an effective hypotensive agent but a significant decrease in resting renin secretion was not found overall (Esler and Nestel, 1973). Surprisingly, these authors also found practolol to reduce urinary noradrenaline output in response to tilting - if confirmed food for thought indeed.

In an early study, Birkenhager et al. (1971) failed to show any correlation between hypotensive action and a fall in renin secretion in 15 hypertensive patients receiving propranolol. Later, however, Buhler et al. (1973) reported that in a study of 96 patients with various forms

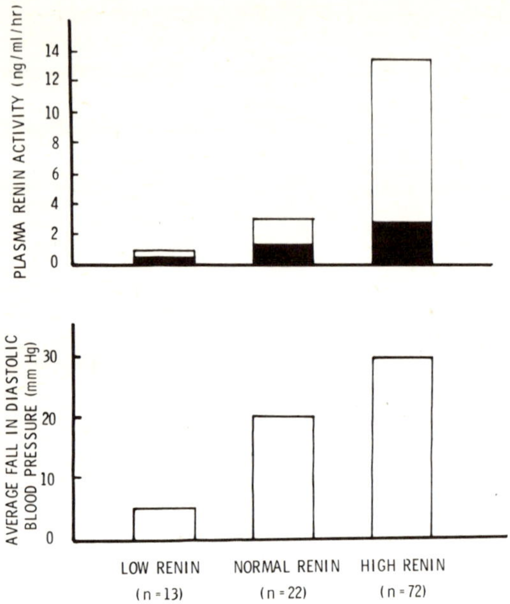

Figure 9.

Relationship between plasma renin values before and after (solid areas) propranolol (average 2 mg/kg/day per os) and the fall in diastolic blood pressure in response to propranolol. (After Buhler et al., 1972).

of hypertension a striking correlation was apparent. Regardless of aetiology, the antihypertensive effectiveness of propranolol correlated with both control renin levels and the decrement in renin secretion. His results are summarized in the illustration and show that the greater effect clearly occurs in the high renin group (Fig. 9). The rapidity of onset is illustrated also where the response of an individual patient with malignant hypertension was both prompt and sustained. Supportive evidence comes from the evaluations of Castenfors et al. (1973) and Hansson et al. (1973) who also show a highly significant correlation between the reduction in systolic pressure and change in plasma renin activity. This suggested causal relationship is questioned by Stokes et al. (1974) who showed that lowering of blood pressure by propranolol was sustained and accompanied by a reduction in renin secretion but that on transference to pindolol, pressure remained low but renin output rose to pre-propranolol levels.

There are clearly many assumptions in this hypothesis, not least the relationship between renin and hypertension or the fact that renin output is more sensitive to propranolol than is hypertension. Nevertheless it has given new life and new paths of thought to an extremely difficult and complex field of study.

HYPERTROPHIC OBSTRUCTIVE CARDIOMYOPATHY

The background to the use of β-blocking agents in this condition has been reviewed by Flamm and Stenson (1971). The symptons of hypertrophic obstructive cardiomyopathy are aggravated by the administration of isoprenaline and by conditions of excessive sympathetic activity such as exercise and excitement. Tissue removed from the outflow tract at surgery contains large amounts of catecholamines. Such considerations suggested that β-adrenoceptor blockade might be of value in decreasing effort-induced obstruction of the outflow tracts. During cardiac catheterization, it was observed that pronethalol decreased the cardiac index and rate of right ventricular pressure development in patients with evidence of this disease and that isoprenaline-induced augmentation of the left ventricular outflow gradients was significantly reduced (Harrison et al., 1964). Similar findings have been reported for propranolol (Cherian et al., 1966) and practolol (Webb-Peploe et al., 1971).

Both in hypertrophic obstructive cardiomyopathy and in tetralogy of Fallot (Cumming, 1970) there appears to be a special dependence on the action of β-adrenoceptor antagonists in cancelling the positive *inotropic* actions of sympathetic neurohormones. This is distinct from most other conditions where the associated oxygen-sparing consequences of negative chronotropic activity may be dominant. Some concern has been expressed at the use of agents with negative inotropic potential in conditions where the predominant symptoms are of left ventricular failure. Hypertrophic cardiomyopathy is characterized by resistance to ventricular filling associated with massive hypertrophy (Stewart et al., 1968). This requires elevated atrial pressure to permit adequate ventricular filling and reduced myocardial contractility under β-adrenergic blockade would only further increase the need for a raised left atrial pressure. This disadvantage would have to be offset by a significant reduction of the left ventricular outflow obstruction to allow any benefit to be obtained. Clinical experience with β-adrenoceptor antagonists in patients with hypertrophic obstructive cardiomyopathy who have symptoms of left ventricular failure indicates that many do show improvement both subjectively and objectively (Adelman et al., 1970; Goodwin, 1970; Stenson et al., 1971).

CONCLUSION

The case has been argued that the primary benefits and associated adverse reactions of β-adrenoceptor antagonists are uniformly linked to the principal pharmacological action i.e. selective inhibition of sympathetic activity whether of neural or circulating hormonal origin. The range of ancillary pharmacological properties are of little, if any, clinical significance. The apparent advantages of cardio-selectivity in terms of a reduced effect on cardiac output may be accepted but have, as yet, no satisfactory explanation.

REFERENCES

Adelman, A.G., Shah, P.M., Gramiak, R. and Wigle, E.D.(1970). Long term propranolol therapy in muscular subaortic stenosis. Brit. Heart J., 32, 804.

Assaykeen, T.A., Clayton, P.L., Goldfien, A. and Ganong, W.F. (1970). The effect of alpha - and beta - adrenergic blocking agents on the renin response to hypoglycaemia and epinephrine in dogs. Endocrinology, 87, 1318.

Assaykeen, T.A. and Ganong, W.F. (1971). The sympathetic nervous system and renin secretion. In: 'Frontiers in Neuroendocrinology'. Eds. Martini, L. and Ganong, W.F. New York : Oxford Univ. Press. p. 67.

Bainbridge, J.G. and Greenwood, D.T. (1971). Tranquillizing effects of propranolol demonstrated in rats. Neuropharmacology, 10, 453.

Bakke, O.M., Davies, D.S., Davies, L. and Dollery, C.T. (1973). Metabolism of propranolol in rat : the fate of the N-isopropyl group. Life Sci., 13, 1665.

Barrett, A.M. (1969). A survey of the pharmacological properties of adrenergic beta-receptor antagonists. Int. J. clin. Pharmac., Suppl. 3, 2.

Barrett, A.M. (1973). The pharmacology of Beta-adrenoceptor antagonists. In 'Recent Advances in Cardiology' 6th ed. Ed. Hamer, J. Edinburgh and London : Churchill Livingstone, p. 289.

Barrett, A.M. and Carter, J. (1970). Comparative chronotropic activity of β-adrenoceptive antagonists. Br. J. Pharmac., 40, 373.

Barrett, A.M. and Cullum, V.A. (1968). The biological properties of the optical isomers of propranolol and their effects on cardiac arrhythmias. Br. J. Pharmac., 34, 43.

Barrett, A. M. and Nunn, B. (1970). Adrenergic neuron blocking properties of (±) - propranolol and (+) -propranolol. J. Pharm. Pharmac., 22, 806.

Barrett, A.M. and Nunn, B. (1971). Intrinsic sympathomimetic activity in relation to the precipitation of heart failure by beta - adrenoceptive blockade. Arch. int. Pharmacodyn., 189, 168.

Birkenhäger, W.H., Krauss, X.H., Schalekamp, M.A.D.H., Kolsters, G. and Kroon, B.U.M. (1971). Antihypertensive effects of propranolol: observations on predictability. *Fol.Med. Neerl.*, **14**, 67.

Black, J.W. and Stephenson, J.S. (1962). Pharmacology of a new adrenergic beta-receptor-blocking compound (nethalide). *Lancet*, **2**, 311.

Brick, I., Hutchinson, K.J., McDevitt, D.G., Roddie, I.C. and Shanks, R.G. (1968). Comparison of the effect of I.C.I. 50172 and propranolol on the cardiovascular responses to adrenaline, isoprenaline and exercise. *Br. J. Pharmac. Chemother.*, **34**, 127.

Bühler, F.R., Laragh, J.H., Baer, L., Vaughan, E.D. and Brunner, H.R. (1972). Propranolol inhibition of renin secretion. *New Engl. J. Med.*, **287**, 1209.

Bühler, F.R., Laragh, J.H., Vaughan, E.D. et al. (1973). Antihypertensive action of propranolol. Specific antirenin responses in high and normal renin forms of essential, renal, renovascular and malignant hypertension. *Am. J. Cardiol.*, **32**, 511.

Burgen, A.S.V. and Iversen, L.L. (1965). The inhibition of noradrenaline uptake by sympathomimetic amines in the rat isolated heart. Br. J. Pharmac. Chemother., 25, 34.

Castenfors, J., Johnsson, H. and Orö, L. (1973). Effect of alprenolol on blood pressure and plasma renin activity in hypertensive patients. Acta med. scand., 193, 189.

Challenor, D.R. and Steinberg, D. (1966a). Effects of free fatty acid on the oxygen consumption of perfused rat heart. Am. J. Physiol., 210, 280.

Challenor, D.R. and Steinberg, D. (1966b). Oxidative metabolism of myocardium as influenced by fatty acids and epinephrine. Am. J. Physiol., 211, 897.

Chamberlain, D.A. (1966a). Effects of beta adrenergic blockade on heart size. Am. J. Cardiol., 18, 321.

Chamberlain, D.A. (1966b). The haemodynamic effect of beta-adrenergic blockade in man. Cardiologia, 49, Suppl. 2, 27.

Cherian, G., Brockington, I.F., Shah, P.M., Oakley, C.M. and Goodwin, J.F. (1966). Beta-adrenergic blockade in hypertrophic obstructive cardiomyopathy. Br. Med. J., 1, 895.

Ciofalo, F., Levitt, B. and Roberts, J. (1967). Some factors affecting ouabain-induced ventricular arrhythmia in the reserpine treated cat. Br. J. Pharmac. Chemother., 30, 143.

Clark, A.J. (1933). The mode of action of drugs on cells. London: Edward Arnold.

Coltart, D.J. (1971). Comparison of effects of propranolol and practolol on exercise tolerance in angina pectoris. Br. Heart J., 33, 62.

Coltart, D.J. and Shand, D.G. (1970). Plasma propranolol levels in the quantitative assessment of beta-adrenergic blockade in man. Br. Med. J., 3, 731.

Conway, E.L. and Lang, W.J. (1974). Cardiovascular responses produced by the injection of isoprenaline and propranolol into the cerebral ventricles of the unanaesthetized dog. Clin. exp. Pharmac. Physiol., 1, 59.

Cumming, G.R. (1970). Beta-adrenergic blockade in paediatric cardiology. In 'Cardiovascular Beta-Adrenergic Responses'. Eds., Kattus, A.A., Ross, G. and Hall, V.E. Los Angeles: Univ. California Press. p. 231.

Dawes, P.M. and Faulkner, D.C. (1974). The effect of propranolol on vascular responses to sympathetic nerve stimulation. Br. J. Pharmac., (in press).

Day, M.D., Owen, D.D.A. and Warren, P.R. (1968). An adrenergic neurone blocking action of propranolol in isolated tissues. J. Pharm. Pharmac., 20, 130S-134S.

Day, M.D. and Roach, A.G. (1973). β-Adrenergic receptors in the central nervous system of the cat concerned with control of arterial blood pressure and heart rate. Nature New Biology, 242, 30.

Dollery, C.T., Lewis, P.J., Myers, M.G. and Reid, J.L. (1973). Central hypotensive effects of propranolol in the rabbit. Br. J. Pharmac., 48, 343P.

Dorph, S. and Binder, C. (1969). Evaluation of the hypotensive effect of beta-adrenergic blockade in hypertension. Acta med. scand., 185, 443.

Dusting, G.J. and Rand, M.J. (1974). An anti-hypertensive action of propranolol in DOCA/salt treated rats. Clin. exp. Pharmac. Physiol., 1, 87.

Eliash, S. and Weinstock, M. (1971). Role of adrenergic neurone blockade in the hypotensive action of propranolol. Br. J. Pharmac., 43, 287.

Esler, M.D. and Nestel, P.J. (1973). Evaluation of practolol in hypertension_ Effects on sympathetic nervous system and renin responsiveness. Br. Heart J., 35, 469.

Fitzgerald, J.D. and Scales, B. (1968). Effect of a new adrenergic beta-blocking agent (ICI 50172) on heart rate in relation to its blood levels. Int. J. Clin. Pharmacol., 1, 467.

Flamm, M.D. and Stenson, R. E. (1971). Beta-adrenergic receptor blockade in hypertrophic subaortic stenosis. In 'Circulatory Effects and Clinical Uses of Beta-Adrenergic Blocking Drugs'. Ed. Harrison, D.C. Amsterdam : Excerpta Medica. p. 96.

Franciosa, J.A., Freis, E.D. and Conway, J. (1973). Anti-hypertensive and haemodynamic properties of the new beta-adrenergic blocking agent timolol. Circulation, 48, 118.

Froloch, E.D., Tarazi, R.C., Dustan, H.P. and Page, I.H. (1968). The paradox of beta-adrenergic blockade in hypertension. Circulation, 37, 417.

Furberg, C. and Michaelson, G. (1969). Effect of 'Aptin', a beta-adrenergic blocking agent, in arterial hypertension. Acta med. scand., 186, 447.

Ganong, W.F. (1973). Biogenic amines, sympathetic nerves and renin secretion. Fed. Proc., 32, 1782.

Ganguly, D.K. and Bhattacharya, B.B. (1970). Adrenergic beta-receptors in vas deferens. Arch. int. pharmacodyn., 185, 406.

Gillam, P.M.S. and Prichard, B.N.C. (1971). Log dose-response curve to assess the effects of propranolol in angina pectoris. Br. J. Pharmac., 41, 408P.

Glaister, D.H., Harrison, M.H. and Allnutt, M.F. (1973). Experimental cardiovascular stress and the influence of oxprenolol. In "New perspectives in beta-blockade". Eds., Burley, D.M., Frier, J.H., Rondel, R.K. and Taylor, S.H. Horsham, England: Ciba Laboratories. p. 241.

Goodwin, J.F. (1970). The role of beta-adrenergic stimulation in obstructive cardiomyopathy and its modification by blocking drugs and surgery. In 'Cardiovascular beta-adrenergic responses'. Eds., Kattus, A.A., Ross, G. and Hall, V.E. Los Angeles: Univ. California Press p. 161.

Grosz, H.J. (1972). Narcotic withdrawal symptoms in heroin users treated with propranolol. Lancet, 2, 564.

Hansson, L. (1973). Beta-adrenergic blockade in essential hypertension. Acta med. scand. Suppl. 550: 1.

Hansson, L., Olander, R. and Åberg, H. (1971). Twice-daily propranolol treatment for hypertension. Lancet, 2, 713.

Harrison, D.C., Braunwald, E., Glick, G., Mason, D.T., Chidsey, C.A. and Ross, J. (1974). Effects of beta-adrenergic blockade on the circulation with particular reference to observations in patients with hypertrophic subaortic stenosis. Circulation, 29, 84.

Hayes, A. and Cooper, R.G. (1971). Studies on the absorption, distribution and excretion of propranolol in rat, dog and monkey. J. Pharmac. exp. ther., 176, 302.

Howe, R. and Shanks, R.G. (1966). Optical isomers of propranolol. Nature, 210, 1336.

Hutter, O.F. and Trautwein, W. (1956). Vagal and sympathetic effects on the pacemaker fibers in the sinus venosus of the heart. J. Gen. Physiol., 39, 715.

Iversen, L.L. (1973). Catecholamine uptake processes. Br. Med. Bull., 29, 130.

Jenkinson, D.H. (1960). The antagonism between tubocurarine and substances which depolarize the motor end-plate. J. Physiol., 152, 309.

Kelliher, G.J. and Buckley, J.P. (1970). Central hypotensive activity of dl- and d-propranolol. J. Pharm. Sci., 59, 1276.

Leishman, A.W.D., Thirkettle, J.L., Allen, B.R. and Dixon, R.A. (1970). Controlled trial of oxprenolol and practolol in hypertension. Br. Med. J., 4, 342.

Leszkovsky, G. and Tardos, L.J. (1965). Some effects of propranolol on the central nervous system. J. Pharm. Pharmac., 17, 518.

Loeffler, J.R., Stockigt, J.R. and Ganong, W.F. (1972). The effect of α- and β-adrenergic blocking agents on the increase in renin secretion produced by stimulation of the renal nerves. Neuroendocrinology, 10, 129.

Lydtin, H., Kusus, T., Daniel, W. et al. (1972). Propranolol therapy in essential hypertension. Am. Heart J., 83, 589.

Masuoka, D. and Hansson, E. (1967). Autoradiographic distribution studies of adrenergic blocking agents. II ^{14}C-propranolol, a β-receptor type blocker. Acta pharmac. tox., 25, 447.

McGibney, D. (1974). Some observations comparing and contrasting the circulatory effects of beta-receptor antagonists with and without cardioselective properties. B.Sc. dissertation. Univ. of Leeds.

Mjøs, O.D. (1971a). Effect of free fatty acids on myocardial function and oxygen consumption in intact dogs. J. clin. Invest., 50, 1386.

Mjøs, O.D. (1971b). Effect of inhibition of lipolysis on myocardial oxygen consumption in the presence of isoproterenol. J. Clin. Invest., 50, 1869.

Morgan, T.O., Louis, W.J., Dawborn, J.K. and Doyle, A.E. (1972). The use of prindolol (Visken) in the treatment of hypertension. Med. J. Aust., 2, 309.

Murmann, W., Almirante, L. and Saccani-Guelfi, M. (1966). Central nervous system effects of four β-adrenergic receptor blocking agents. J. Pharm. Pharmac., 18, 317.

Mylecharane, E.J. and Raper, C. (1970). Prejunctional actions of some β-adrenoceptor antagonists in the vas deferens preparation of the guinea pig. Br. J. Pharmac., 39, 128.

Mylecharane, E.J. and Raper, C. (1973). Further studies on the adrenergic neuron blocking activity of some β-adrenoceptor antagonists and guanethidine. J. Pharm. Pharmac., 25, 213.

Norman, J. and Whitwam, J.G. (1974). Modification by atropine and practolol of changes in heart rate evoked by cutaneous nerve stimulation. Br. J. Pharmac., 51, 150P.

Passo, S.S., Assaykeen, T.A., Goldfien, A. and Ganong, W.F. (1971). Effect of α- and β-adrenergic blocking agents on the increase in renin secretion produced by stimulation of the medulla oblongata in dogs. Neuroendocrinology, 7, 97.

Paterson, J.W., Conolly, M.E., Dollery, C.T., Hayes, A. and Cooper R.G. (1970). The pharmacodynamics and metabolism of propranolol in man. Pharmacologia clin., 2, 127.

Paton, W.D.M. and Payne, J.P. (1968). Pharmacological principles and practice. London: Churchill.

Prichard, B.N.C. (1964). Hypotensive action of pronethalol. Br. Med. J., 1, 1227.

Prichard, B.N.C. (1971). Aspects of the evaluation of antihypertensive drugs. Arch. int. pharmacodyn., 192, Suppl. p. 193.

Prichard, B.N.C., Aellig, W.H. and Richardson, G.A. (1970). The action of intravenous oxprenolol, practolol, propranolol and sotalol on acute exercise tolerance in angina pectoris. Postgrad. med. J., 46, Suppl. p. 77.

Prichard, B.N.C., Dickinson, C.J., Alleyne, G.A.O., Hurst, P., Hill, I.D., Rosenheim, M.L. and Laurence, D.R. (1963). Effect of pronethalol in angina pectoris. Br. Med. J., 2, 1226.

Prichard, B.N.C. and Gillam, P.M.S. (1964). Use of propranolol (Inderal) in treatment of hypertension. Br. Med. J., 2, 725.

Prichard, B.N.C. and Gillam, P.M.S. (1969). Treatment of hypertension with propranolol. Br. Med. J., 1, 7.

Reid, I.A., Stockigt, J.A., Goldfien, A. and Ganong, W.F. (1972). Stimulation of renin secretion in dogs by theophylline. Europ. J. Pharmac., 17, 325.

Reid, J.L., Lewis, P.J., Myers, M.G. and Dollery, C.T. (1974). Cardiovascular effects of intracerebroventricular d-, l- and dl propranolol in the conscious rabbit. J. Pharmac. exp. Ther., 188, 394.

Robinson, B.F. (1971). The mode of action of beta-antagonists in angina pectoris. Postgraduate Med. J., 47, Suppl. p. 41.

Scales, B. and Cosgrove, M.B. (1970). The metabolism and distribution of the selective adrenergic beta-blocking agent, practolol. J. Pharmac. exp. Ther., 175, 338.

Simpson, F. O. and Waal-Manning, H.J. (1970). Hypertension and β-adrenergic blockade. In: 'New Horizons in Medicine (1)'. Sydney: Sandoz. p. 59.

Sommerville, W., Taggart, P. and Carruthers, M. (1971). Addressing a medical meeting: effect on heart rate, electrocardiogram, plasma catecholamines, free fatty acids and triglycerides. Br. Heart J., 33, 608.

Stenson, R.E., Flamm, M.D., Harrison, D.C. and Hancock, E.W. (1973). Hypertrophic subaortic stenosis: clinical and haemodynamic effects of long term propranolol therapy. Am. J. Cardiol., 31, 763.

Stewart, S., Mason, D.T. and Braunwald, E. (1968). Impaired rate of left ventricular filling in idiopathic hypertrophic subaortic stenosis and valvular aortic stenosis. Circulation, 37, 8.

Stokes, G.S., Weber, M.A. and Thornell, I.R. (1974). β-Blockers and plasma renin activity in hypertension. Br. Med. J., 1, 60.

Taggart P. and Carruthers, M. (1971). Endogenous hyperlipidaemia induced by emotional stress of racing driving. Lancet, 1, 363.

Taggart, P. and Carruthers, M. (1972). Suppression by oxprenolol of adrenergic response to stress. Lancet, 2, 256.

Taggart, P., Gibbons, D. and Sommerville, W. (1969). Some effects of motor car driving on the normal and abnormal heart. Br. Med. J., 4, 130.

Tarazi, R.C. and Dustan, H.P. (1972). Beta adrenergic blockade in hypertension. Practical and theoretical implications of long term hemodynamic variations. Am. J. Cardiol., 29, 633.

Taylor, S.H. (1973). Mechanism of action of adrenergic beta-receptor antagonists in angina pectoris. In 'New perspectives in beta-blockade'. Eds. Burley, D.M., Frier, J.H., Rondel, R.K. and Taylor, S.H. Horsham, England: Ciba Laboratories. p. 107.

Thadani, U., Sharma, B., Meeran, M.K., Majid, P.A., Whitaker, W. and Taylor, S.H. (1973). Comparison of adrenergic beta-receptor antagonists in angina pectoris. Br. Med. J., 1, 138.

Tindell, G.L., Walle, T. and Gaffney, T.E. (1972). Rat liver microsomal metabolism of propranolol: identification of seven metabolites by gas chromatography - mass spectrometry. Life Sci., 11, 1029.

Tobert, J.A., Slater, J.D.H., Fogelman, F., Lightman, S.L., Kurtz., A.B. and Payne, N.N. (1973). The effect in man of (+)-propranolol and racemic propranolol on renin secretion stimulated by orthostatic stress. Clin. Sci., 44, 291.

Tsien, R.W. (1973). Adrenaline-like effects of intracellular iontophoresis of cyclic-AMP in cardiac Purkinje fibres. Nature New Biology, 245, 120.

Ulrych, M., Frolich, E.D., Dustan, H.P. and Page, I.H. (1968). Immediate hemodynamic effects of beta-adrenergic blockade with propranolol in normotensive and hypertensive men. Circulation, 37, 411.

Vaughan Williams, E.M. (1970). Classification of anti-arrhythmic drugs. In Symposium on Cardiac Arrhythmias. Eds. Sandøe, E., Flensted-Jensen, E. and Olesen, K.H. Södertälje, Sweden: A.B. Astra.

Walle, T., Ishizaki, T. and Gaffney, T.E. (1972). Isopropylamine, a biologically active deamination product of propranolol in dogs. J. Pharmac. exp. Ther., 183, 508.

Webb-Peploe, M.M., Croxson, R.S., Oakley, C.M. and Goodwin, J.F. (1971). Cardioselective beta-adrenergic blockade in hypertrophic obstructive myopathy. Postgrad. Med. J., 47, Suppl. p. 93.

Weber, M.A., Thornell, I.R. and Stokes, G.S. (1972). Differing effects of the three β-blocking agents on plasma renin activity in the conscious rabbit.

Widerøe, T.E. and Vigander, T. (1974). Propranolol in the treatment of migraine, Br. Med. J., 2, 699.

Wilson, A.G., Brooke, O.G., Lloyd, H.J. and Robinson, B.F. (1969). Mechanism of action of β-adrenergic receptor blocking agents in angina pectoris: comparison of action of propranolol with dexpropranolol and practolol. Br. Med. J., 4, 399.

Zacharias, F.J., Cowen, R.J., Prestt, J., Vickers, J. and Wall, B.G. (1972). Propranolol in hypertension. A long term study of therapy 1964-1970. Am. Heart J., 83, 755.